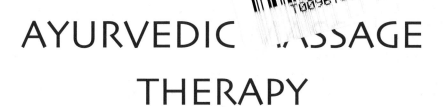

AYURVEDIC MASSAGE THERAPY

THERAPY

BY

Dr. Subhash Ranade

Dr. Rajan Rawat

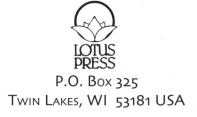

LOTUS
PRESS
P.O. Box 325
Twin Lakes, WI 53181 USA

This book is dedicated to all students and practitioners of Ayurveda. It is our sincere wish that it enriches your knowledge of this wonderful system of healing and health.

DISCLAIMER

Edited by David Freedman

Copyright © 2008   Dr. Subhash Ranade & Dr. Rajan Rawat

First Edition October 2008

Printed in the United States of America

ISBN   978-0-9409-8599-5

Library of Congress Catalog Number   2007939776

Published by:
Lotus Press, P.O. Box 325, Twin Lakes, WI 53181 USA
web: www.lotuspress.com
Email: lotuspress@lotuspress.com
800.824.6396

CONTENTS

PREFACE

Massage is an ancient Indian art used for healing and relaxation as well as for treating various diseases. The touch of massage can bring about dramatic changes in the body and mind. Ayurvedic massage has many unique features and advantages versus any other oriental or modern system of massage.

Ayurvedic massage is done according to body constitution, age, stage of the disease, aggravated doshas, status of agni and ama. With this understanding, the Ayurvedic masseur can choose the correct type of oil or other substances for massage, bringing about dramatic results for both healthy as well as diseased patients.

In spite of the development of sophisticated equipment for treating various physical injuries and a wide range of electrical apparatus, it is quite surprising that if one understands the fundamental principles of Ayurveda, and the correct oil or substance and methods are used, much better results can be found.

Many authors have written about Ayurvedic massage. However, very few have given proper consideration to the basic principles of Ayurveda. Therefore, while writing this book, we have explained the fundamental principles of Ayurveda in the first chapters. Later on we have explained various methods, as well as oils and other substances used for massage.

For the first time we have explained the very important concept of "Marma massage" which is becoming very popular not only in India, but also abroad. The chapter on "Massage for Specific Diseases" has highlighted some important diseases in which massage can be very useful.

The authors are thankful to Dr. Ajit Mandalecha for providing valuable material and helpful suggestions.

We wish to also mention the efforts taken by David Freedman who is one of my students from the AYU Ayurvedic Academy, directed by Dr. Vivek Shanbhag. David has taken a lot of effort in the editing of this book, including rewriting many concepts and rephrasing them so that the entire matter will be user friendly to Western readers. He has devoted many months of his valuable time and we have no words to thank him.

We hope that this book will receive a good response from the Ayurvedic as well as other scientific communities.

Dr. Subhash Ranade
Rajbharati, 367 Sahakar Nagar 1
Pune, India411, 009
sbranade@rediffmail.com

Dr. Rajan Rawat
'Shri' 38,Shamsundar Hsg. Soc,
Pune, India 411,030
drrajan_rawat@hotmail.com

INTRODUCTION

Ayurveda is the traditional medicine of India. It has a very long history, having been practiced continually for over 5,000 years. Having existed for such a long time, Ayurveda is not just a medical system, it is an integral part of Indian culture. Massage is one of many techniques used in Ayurveda for both treatment and prevention of disease. In this book you will find specialized Ayurvedic massage techniques, lists of therapeutic oils and treatments for specific diseases using Ayurvedic massage. The section on self massage is important as daily self massage can prevent many health disorders.

We have explained some of the main concepts of Ayurvedic medical theory including a questionnaire to help determine your particular body type, which is a main focus of Ayurvedic practice. English translations are used whenever possible, with Ayurvedic terms following in parenthesis. Many quotations from classical textbooks have been included. These are followed by abbreviations such as Su (Sushruta), Ch (Charaka), AH (Ashtanga Hridaya), etc. A listing of these classical texts and the abbreviations used can be found near the end of the book.

For those with a background in Ayurveda, differences may be noted from other books or teaching in regard to explanation of certain concepts and techniques. This is common in Oriental medicine and is usually due to different interpretations and schools that have evolved over a long period of time.

As you read through the book you may find spellings that are slightly different than you have seen before. This is part of the rich culture of India where there are currently in use 29 different languages and 300 different dialects. An example is the common replacement of letters in words. This changes sattva to sattwa, basti to vasti, marma to varma or Prakruti to Prakriti. The spelling is different, but the meaning is still the same.

We hope that you find this book both interesting and useful and that it enriches both your life and the lives of others.

CHAPTER 1

HISTORY OF MASSAGE

A word for massage exists in almost every culture. Massage is perhaps the most popular form of health activity today. It is effectively used for achieving relaxation and as a form of natural therapy for various diseases. The art of massage has been practiced since ancient times and in many countries. Early physicians used massage effectively in treating fatigue, illness and injury. Studies of classical texts indicate that the ancient Chinese, Greeks and Romans all practiced a form of massage. Roman and Greek philosophers and physicians prescribed massage not only for its restorative powers after battle, but for general health of the body and mind. The ancient Greeks established massage schools in their gymnasiums and used massage for maintaining health as well as for treating various diseases. The famous Greek poet Homer mentions beautiful girls giving massage to the fatigued soldiers who returned from war.

In the Far East, the Indian cultures and their epic texts like Ramayana and Mahabharata describe massage for health maintenance. The Bhavishya Purana, which is a very ancient text, mentions different techniques of massage. These techniques include how a wife should give massage to her husband, both for health benefits and for increasing sexual power and enjoyment. In India, performing musicians and actors learn massage practices to aid their artistic development. In the book Vatsyayana Kamasutra, massage has been explained for the purpose of enhancing sexual power. This text mentions three different types of massage. Samvahana (whole body massage), keshamardana (head massage) and utsadana (massage done to the feet). The text has described the art of massage as one of the 64 Kalas (arts), which also include music, dance, poetry and drama.

In some societies massage has been used socially as an act of hospitality, as in Hawaii, where passive movements called Lomi-Lomi are bestowed on honored guests. This is a traditional massage of Hawaii and gives relaxation to all the muscles in the body.

In Ayurveda there are three main text books, known as the bruhat trayi, which in Sanskrit means "big triad" or "big three". These are the Charaka samhita, Sushruta samhita and the Ashtang Hridaya. These texts give detailed explanations of the use of massage in prevention and treatment. These three texts are still used today in university level Ayurveda courses. Along with the "bruhat trayi", the technique of massage has been explained in texts such as the yogratnakara and bhavaprakasha. In 18th century India, massage was regularly given to sportsman as well as to soldiers.

Massage has also become very popular in Europe due to the work of Per Henrik Ling of Sweden. After a visit to China to study massage, Ling developed his own method of massage which became known throughout the world as Swedish massage. Later on, in the 19th century, two separate branches of massage, physiotherapy and occupational therapy came into existence.

CHAPTER 2

BASIC PRINCIPLES OF AYURVEDA

Ayurveda is one of the great gifts of the sages of ancient India to mankind. It is one of the oldest scientific medical systems in the world, with a long record of clinical experience to validate it. However, it is not just a system of medicine in the conventional sense of curing disease. It is also a way of life that teaches us how to maintain and protect health. It shows us how to both cure disease and how to promote health and longevity. Ayurveda treats man as a "whole", though at the same time viewing him as a combination of body, mind and soul. Ayurveda is truly a holistic and integral medical system.

The word "Ayu" means all aspects of life from birth to death. The word "Veda" means knowledge or learning. Thus "Ayurveda" denotes the science by which life in its totality is understood. It is a science of life that delineates the diet, medicines and behavior that are beneficial or harmful for life.

Ayurveda is said to have originated in the very beginning of the cosmic creation. Indian philosophers state that Ayurveda originates from Brahma, the creator of the universe. Brahma is not a mere individual but the unmanifest form of the Divine Lord, from whom the whole manifest world has come into being. The desire to keep fit, healthy and live long is found in the basic instincts of each organism. In this respect Ayurveda is the paradigm for other systems of medicine. Ayurveda is a tradition with an antiquity concurrent with that of life itself.

Ayurveda accepts the concept of a common origin of the universe and man. The universe is the macrocosm, while man is the microcosm. For the creation of the universe two types of substances are essential: material and non-material.

Trigunas - Super qualities

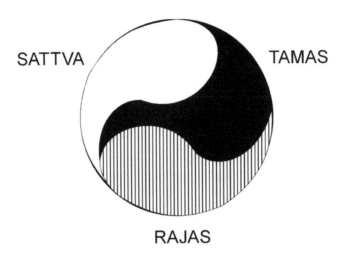

SATTVA TAMAS

RAJAS

Trigunas

Guna means attribute or quality. In Ayurveda there is a concept of the three gunas, referred to as the trigunas. The trigunas are the three ultimate qualities at work in nature which are behind all material forms. The three gunas are referred to as Sattva, Rajas and Tamas. Sattva is consciousness or knowledge. Rajas is motion or action. Tamas is the inertia resisting Sattva and Rajas. For the creation of any substance in the universe the contribution of these three non-material substances is essential.

Five Element Theory/Quantum physics - Panchamahabhutas

The five basic material elements that exist in the universe and in man are called the five great elements (Pancha Mahabhutas). Pancha means five and Mahabhutas means great elements. These five elements are space - also referred to as ether - (akasha), air (vayu), fire (tejas), water (apa) and earth (prithvi). Space is the area in which all things are manifested. Air is responsible for all motion. Fire is the energy or heat which makes all transformation possible. Water is the liquid form in the universe and Earth is the solid mass. These five elements are the principles of density that apply to all manifested forms, including the mind. These five elements range in density from space, which is completely subtle, allowing total freedom and action, to Earth which is completely dense and which allows no action. Between these two polarities are all possible densities and forms.

Basic element	Sanskrit term	Form or action
SPACE	akasha	SPACE
AIR	vayu	MOTION
FIRE	tejas	ENERGY/HEAT
WATER	apa or jala	LIQUID
EARTH	prithvi	SOLID MASS

When these five basic elements in the Universe are in balance, all activity occurs in its proper balance and order. When these five basic elements become out of balance, natural calamities occur such as floods, cyclones or earthquakes, along with extremes of heat and cold. In human beings, if these five basic elements are in the proper balance we are healthy. When they are imbalanced all types of disorders can take place.

If there is an excess of the element of space in the body, which forms the hollow spaces, there is an increase in deformities like cavities in the lungs, or osteoporosis, an increase in the hollowness of the bones. When the space element gets decreased, solid tumors and hypertrophy of the organs takes place. An excess of the element of air, which controls movement in the body, may cause tremors or tachycardia, an increased heart rate, (tachycardia can also be caused by an increase in the fire element). When there is a decrease in air we see paresis, paralysis or improper movement of muscles. An excess of fire in the body can cause inflammations, fevers or ulcers. A decrease in the fire element, and the resulting low digestive fire, may result in indigestion. With an excess accumulation of water in the body, deformities like edema, pleurisy or ascites can take place, while because of its decrease, dehydration can occur. With excess of earth, solid tumors or obesity can occur, while due to its decrease there may be loss of weight.

CHAPTER 3

AYURVEDIC ANATOMY

Various older Ayurvedic texts have described in detail the number and descriptions of the bones, joints, ligaments, muscles, tendons, veins and arteries. During that era, the method of dissecting bodies was different from that of today, and the description and numbers of these body parts may differ from modern textbooks of anatomy. More importantly however, is the accuracy in which the function of the various organs and systems has been explained in the ancient texts.

The Ayurvedic surgeon and author Sushruta, has explained the organs and structures in detail as follows.

1. Bones (asthi) - 300

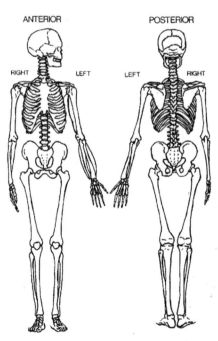

Skeleton

Modern anatomy has described 206 bones, while in Ayurveda all the cartilages have been included under bones. These can be classified into bones proper, cartilages, teeth and nails.

LOCATION	NUMBER
EXTREMITIES	120
TRUNK	117
HEAD AND NECK	63
TOTAL	300

Our bones are known collectively as the skeleton, which means "dried up". Contrary to their appearance after death, they are extremely dynamic and versatile structures, which protect important organs and give support and strength to the body.

Joints (sandhi)

EXTREMITIES	68
TRUNK	59
HEAD AND NECK	83
TOTAL	210

The bony joints have been divided into three types; movable, partially movable and non-movable.

a. Moveable -
- hinge joints (kora) - such as the knee and elbow
- ball and socket (ulukhala) - hip and shoulder
b. Partially moveable -
- saddle joints (samudga) - sacro iliac and clavicle
- the joints in between vertebrae (pratara)
- opening like the beak of a bird (vayastunda) - temporomandibular
c. Non-moveable -
- joints in the skull bones (tunna sevani)

Ligaments (snayu) - 900
These are the sub tissues which bind the bones and muscles (Su. sh. 5/42). They are of 4 types. Ligaments, tendons, sphincter muscles and apponeurosis.

LOCATION	NUMBER
EXTREMITIES	600
TRUNK	230
HEAD AND NECK	70
TOTAL	900
MUSCLES (PESHI) -	500

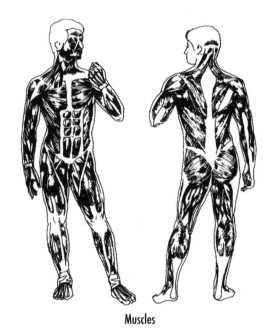

Muscles

LOCATION	NUMBER
EXTREMITIES	400
TRUNK	66
HEAD AND NECK	34
TOTAL	500

When muscle tissue forms different shapes due to the action of Vata, it is referred to as peshi.

a. Bahala - large muscles like biceps and triceps.

b. Pelava - very small muscles, such as those around the metacarpal or metatarsal bones of the hands and feet, which originate from the carpal tunnels.

c. Sthoola - very big, such as the muscles on the buttocks (gluteus major).

d. Anu - extremely small, such as the muscles in the eyeball.

e. Pruthu - big, flat muscles as on the chest (pectoralis major).

f. Vrutta - round shaped, such as the muscles over the shoulder joint (deltoid).

g. Kathina - the hard muscles on the thighs (quadriceps).

h. Mrudu - the soft muscles around the eye (orbicularis oculi).

i. Deergha - the long muscles from the shoulder joint to the arm (pronator longus).

j. Rooksha - rough muscles, such as those in the large intestines.

k. Hrasva - short muscles, such as those in the wrist joint.

Muscles are everywhere in our body. Muscles record our feelings, and their tensions help ease stressful situations. However, when this tension is not released sufficiently the lining of the muscles and the surrounding tissues become irritated, resulting in fibrositis

Tendons (kandara) - 16

LOCATION	NUMBER
EXTREMITIES	8
TRUNK	4
HEAD AND NECK	4
TOTAL	16

Vessels (sira) - 700 (this includes veins and arteries).

In many Ayurvedic texts sira refers to veins and arteries. However, this explanation is not complete. Sira is more broadly defined as channels supplying water or energy to the field or body. Sushruta has explained 4 types of sira. Various experts have tried to correlate these structures with some modern anatomical structures, however their explanation is not satisfactory. Still it is certain that these are channels (srotas), which carry vital fluids or energy to the entire body.

Nerves (dhamani) -

Some authors have explained that the word dhamani means nerves. However, there are other interpretations. The Ashtanga Sangraha text has used the word Vata vaha for nerves. Most of the Yogic texts use the word nadi for nerves. The Shiva Samhita explains that there are 350,000 nerves or nadis. The Siddha medical system accepts the number of nadis as 72,000.

The Skin

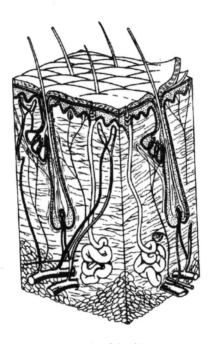

Structure of the Skin

The skin is a very important structure in regard to massage. It is related with various doshas, subdoshas and channels (srotas when singular, srotamsi when plural). In the ancient period of Sushruta and Charaka, although instruments such as microscopes were not available, both authors described 7 and 6 layers of the skin respectively and the diseases that originate from each of these layers. Sushruta has given names to all the 7 layers while Charaka has given names only to the first 2 layers.

Skin Anatomy/ Physiology

- ## Layers of Skin

Sushruta 7 layers
1. Avabhasini—Sidhma kushtha
2. Lohita —Moles
3. Sheta —Charmadala
4. Tamra —Erysepelas
5. Vedini —Leprosy
6. Rohini —Elephantitis
7. Mamsadhara —Abscess, fistula----

Charaka 6 Layers
Udakadhara —Rasa
Asrugdhara —Rakta
Third —Mamsa
Fourth—Meda
Fifth—Majja
Sixth—Deeper vessels

Layer 1. (avabhasini) - This first layer is connected with the skin and plasma (rasa). Charaka has named this layer as udakadhara. This can be compared to the modern term stratum cornium. Sidhma kushtha, a type of skin disease originates from this layer.

Layer 2. (lohita) - Asrugdhara - This second layer is the seat of the blood vessels (rakta) This can be compared to the modern term stratum lucidium. Moles are located in this layer.

Layer 3. (shweta) - This third layer is the location of the muscles (mamsa). This layer is the seat of charmadala type of skin disease. The modern term for this layer is stratum granulosum.

Layer 4. (tamra) - This is the forth layer and is the seat of fatty tissue (meda) which is connected with diseases like erysipelas or vitiligo. (stratum spinosum).

Layer 5. (vedini) - The fifth layer is the seat of nerve endings (stratum basale).

Layer 6. (rohini) - The sixth layer is connected with deeper blood vessels and lymph vessels (papillary and reticular region).

Layer 7. (mamsadhara) - The seventh layer is the seat of sweat glands. All types of abscesses, fistula, etc. take place in this layer only. (subcutaneous layer).

The skin is related with the channels of water metabolism, plasma, blood, fatty tissue, muscular tissue and nervous tissue. The optimum quality, referred to as sara in Ayurveda, of plasma has been explained in the ancient texts as Tvak Sara. Tvak which means skin. This shows that plasma is very closely related to the skin.

Although the skin is connected with all the tridosha, one can say that prana and vyana types of Vata, bhrajaka Pitta and kledaka Kapha are closely related with the skin (see chapter 4 for explanation of dosha subtypes).

The function of sweat is to eliminate the moisture attribute of the subtle waste product (kleda). Kledaka kapha protects the skin from external dryness and heat in the same way that kledaka kapha protects the stomach lining. Oils that are applied for the purpose of massage and various ointments are absorbed by the skin through the action of bhrajaka Pitta along with Vata dosha. Gentle and soothing touch to the skin calms the nerves and the mind and can produce an excellent relaxing effect.

CHAPTER 4

AYURVEDIC PHYSIOLOGY

The Three Biological Humors -Tridosha

There are three main causative factors in the external universe: the sun, the moon, and the wind (or movement). The sun, or the energy of conversion, is represented by fire. The moon, or agency of cooling and interlinking, is represented by the combination of earth and water. Wind, the principle of propulsion or movement, is represented by a combination of air and space (space is also referred to as ether). All natural phenomena observed in the universe are caused by one of these three energies.

1) the energy of propulsion and movement
2) the energy of interchanging/transformation
3) the energy of cohesion.

Vata

The energy of propulsion or movement causes a change in position of all things in the Universe, such as dust, smoke and clouds. In human beings, the functions such as respiration, circulation and elimination (the expulsion of waste products) are manifested as changes in position. This energy of propulsion which is referred to as the biological air humor, is called Vata meaning "that which moves things". Vata is the motivating force behind the other two bodily humors or energies Pitta and Kapha, which are considered to be lame without the influence of Vata. It is said that if you control Vata, you control all disease.

Pitta

Pitta is the biological fire humor and means "that which digests things". When any substance comes in contact with the heat of the Sun, its temperature, form, appearance or taste is changed. In the human body the same thermogenic energy transforms the ingested food into tissues and waste products.

The energy of transformation or conversion is known as Pitta. This energy is through the action of Agni, which is the digestive fire. Agni works through the medium of various hot secretions which are a function of Pitta. Although Pitta is not Agni, the two are intimately related.

Kapha

Kapha is the biological water humor and means "that which holds things together." The effects of the energies of Vata and Pitta are inhibited by Kapha, the energy of cold and cohesion, which in nature produces rainfall. This force is responsible for new growth in the body

DOSHA	MAIN FUNCTION
Vata	Propulsion/movement
Pitta	Transformation/conversion
Kapha	Cohesion/growth

These three primary life forces, or energies, Vata, Pitta and Kapha, are referred to as biological humors, or energies, and are called doshas in the Sanskrit language The science of these three humors is referred to as tridosha. These humors, or energies, are very subtle substances and are the primary forces behind all physiological and psychological functions in the body.

Properties of tridosha

Each dosha has a defined set of properties or qualities. Vata is recognized by its qualities of dry, light, mobile, agitated, cool, rough, less- nourishing, propulsive and subtle. It possesses an astringent taste. When the living body comes into contact with substances of similar qualities, it loses bodily constituents. Even though these qualities are harmful to existing tissues in the body, they are essential for body functions. If these qualities in the structure of a tissue are missing, there will be no movement in it at all.

Pitta is slightly oily, sharp with an unpleasant odor, light, and fluidic (liquid, flowing in some direction) with secretory and vasodilating properties. It has penetrating and hot qualities, and is pungent and sour in taste. In the process of digestion it is an easily flowing fluid. All colors except white and dusky or violet denote existence of Pitta.

Kapha is wet, oily, cool, smooth, sticky, dull, heavy, nourishing, slimy, compact (dense), white in color and both sweet and salty by taste.

VATA	PITTA	KAPHA
cold	hot	cold
dry	slightly oily	oily
rough	smooth	smooth
light	light	heavy
moving	flowing	stable
subtle	penetrating	gross

The underlined qualities in the table above, such as cold, are similar in both Vata and Kapha. Oily is similar in both Pitta and Kapha, and light is similar in both Vata and Pitta. These similarities, along with the differences, become important when determining treatment plans, especially for dual constitutions such as pitta-kapha, vata-kapha or vata-pitta. The similarities and differences are also important in treating dual diseases where more than one dosha is out of balance.

Functions of the Doshas

Functions of Vata

Vata, as the principle of propulsion, carries out many diverse functions in the human body. It controls cell division and arrangement of cells and their formation in different layers. It conducts afferent impulses from special sensory organs (Jnanendriyas) to the brain and efferent impulses from the brain to motor organs (Karmendriyas). Vata controls the expulsion of feces, urine, sweat, menstrual fluid, semen and the fetus. It also controls the respiratory, cardiac and gastro-intestinal movements, as well as all higher functions in the brain and spinal cord. Vata controls the mind and gives us the energy to perform all bodily activities, subtle and gross, as well as mental activity.

Functions of Pitta

Pitta is responsible for the formation of tissues (dhatu), waste products (malas) and energy (doshas) from the food, water and air that we take in from the outside. Pitta controls our metabolic activity, both anabolic, which is building, and catabolic, which is breaking down. It is responsible for all the secretions in the gastro-intestinal tract along with the enzymes and hormones from the ductless glands that enter the blood stream. It controls body temperature as well. Sensations of hunger, thirst, anger and lust are all controlled by Pitta. Pitta is also responsible for actions of bravery and the assimilation of all knowledge from the outside.

Functions of Kapha

Kapha increases the deposits in the cell mass, protects all the tissues in the body from wear and tear and maintains the strength and immunity of the body. The capacity for reproduction, zest, and correct retention of knowledge depends upon the proper function of Kapha. Kapha is essential for the cohesion and interlinking of cells, tissues and organs and is thus responsible for the growth of the body.

Sub Types of Vata, Pitta and Kapha

Sub Types of Vata

THE FIVE FORMS OF VATA

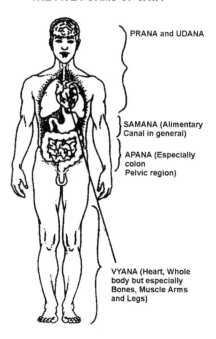

PRANA and UDANA

SAMANA (Alimentary
Canal in general)

APANA (Especially
colon
Pelvic region)

VYANA (Heart, Whole
body but especially
Bones, Muscle Arms
and Legs)

Each dosha has five subtypes. The five subtypes of Vata are Prana, Udana, Vyana, Samana and Apana.

1. Prana - 2. Udana

Prana and Udana are exactly opposite movements. Although the function of Prana can be studied at the level of the brain, heart and lungs, generally speaking its movement is from outside to within and forward. Pranic propulsion is responsible for receiving substances like air, water, food and knowledge from the outside world through the five sense organs.

Udana propulsion is from the inside to the outside and upward, mainly as expiration. Speech is due to Udana, and remembrance is the bringing out of knowledge that has been put in by the Prana.

3. Vyana - 4. Samana

Vyana is located in the heart. It is responsible for both the movement of the heart and the propulsion of nutritive substances in the body. Vyana is also responsible for the movement of the limbs and the flow of the blood and sweat.

Samana is located in the small intestine and is responsible for the movement of food through the stomach and intestines. Samana is involved in digestion through the propulsion of digestive fluids into the small intestine, as well as in the separation of food into nutritive and non-nutritive parts. After digestion in the small intestine samana moves the food into the colon.

5. Apana

In contrast to the two pairs above, the function of apana is to control the movements of constituents like urine, feces, menstrual discharge, seminal discharge and flatus. All these are controlled for a particular period of time before being discharged from the body. The overall control of all these substances for such a period is beneficial to building or maintaining the tissues. Since this control is beneficial to other types of Vata, it is said that Apana controls the different forms of Vata

Sub Types of Pitta

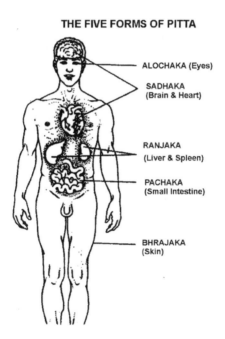

THE FIVE FORMS OF PITTA

ALOCHAKA (Eyes)

SADHAKA
(Brain & Heart)

RANJAKA
(Liver & Spleen)

PACHAKA
(Small Intestine)

BHRAJAKA
(Skin)

The five sub types of Pitta are Pachaka, Ranjaka, Alochaka, Sadhaka and Bhrajaka. All of these are responsible for some type of digestion or conversion.

1. Pachaka

Pachaka is located in the stomach and small intestines and is responsible for the primary conversion of food in the gastro-intestinal tract. It is responsible for conversion of the elements in the food to the bodily elements. Because of its hot and penetrating quality it disintegrates and digests food in the gastro-intestinal tract.

2. Ranjaka

Ranjaka is located in the liver and helps in the secondary digestion of food for the formation of tissues. The formation of blood (rakta) and all other tissues is the chief function of Ranjaka Pitta. Ranjaka works in close association with the tissue fires (dhatu agnis) and elemental fires (bhuta agnis), i.e. space, air, fire, water and earth.

3. Alochaka

There are two types of Alochaka Pitta. The first type is located in the eyes and is responsible for the conversion that takes place when an object is being sensed by the eye. This is observed in the mechanism responsible for photosensation The second type of Alochaka Pitta is responsible for the conversion involved in the sense organs of the ear, the tongue and the nose.

4. Sadhaka

Sadhaka is located in the brain. After sensing an object, its real and quick understanding (comprehension) is dependent upon a specific sequence of conversions by Sadhaka Pitta. The capacity of creative art is a function of Sadhaka Pitta.

5. Bhrajaka

Bhrajaka is located in the skin and is responsible for the digestion and conversion of oils and ointments applied to the skin. Bhrajaka also maintains the temperature and complexion of the skin.

Sub Types of Kapha

THE FIVE FORMS OF KAPHA

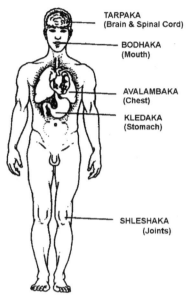

TARPAKA
(Brain & Spinal Cord)

BODHAKA
(Mouth)

AVALAMBAKA
(Chest)

KLEDAKA
(Stomach)

SHLESHAKA
(Joints)

The five sub types of Kapha are Avalambaka, Kledaka, Bodhaka, Tarpaka, and Shleshaka. All of these protect various body parts from wear and tear due to Vata and the hot and penetrating effects of Pitta. Similarly, they help in the cohesion and interlinking of tissues.

1. Avalambaka

Avalambaka is located in the lungs, heart, vertebral column and pelvic girdle and gives protection to them. Due to repeated contraction and relaxation, the lungs and heart are subjected to substantial wear and tear. The fine slimy and oily secretions due to avalambaka inside these organs protects and maintains their integrity.

2. Kledaka

Kledaka is located in the stomach and intestines and protects the upper and middle abdomen from hot, irritating or cold food and drinks as well as from the secretions of Pachaka Pitta.

3. Bodhaka

Bodhaka is located in the mouth and protects the mouth from pungent, hot, cold, or irritating food and drinks. It is responsible for experiencing the various tastes of food. Bodhaka guards the body by initially rejecting potentially harmful substances put into the mouth.

4. Shleshaka

Shleshaka is located in all the joints in the body. It lubricates the bony ends of the joints and protects them from friction during movement.

5. Tarpaka

Tarpaka is located in the brain and spinal chord. It provides various nutrients to the brain cells and gives lubrication and protection to the brain and spinal cord.

Tissues (Dhatus)

The tissues (dhatus) are the constituents in the body which do not get eliminated (except the reproductive), and they remain well within a particular limit. This limit is the skin from the outside of the body, and the internal linings of the gastro-intestinal tract, bladder, joints, cerebral linings, etc., from within the body. There are seven tissues (dhatus).

1. Plasma (rasa)
2. Blood (rakta)
3. Muscle (mamsa)
4. Adipose tissue/fat (meda)
5. Bone (asthi)
6. Bone marrow and nerve tissue (majja)
7. Reproductive tissue (shukra)

Functions of the Tissues

1. Plasma (rasa) provides nutrition to all tissues and gives a sense of pleasure, happiness and contentment. It is responsible for hydration of the tissues and maintaining the electrolyte balance of the body. One of the meanings of the term rasa is "to circulate".
2. Blood (rakta) is the particulate matter in the blood, meaning the red and white blood cells, platelets, etc. Apart from giving Prana or vital force (oxygenation) to all tissues, it is also responsible for love and faith. The term rakta means "to give color".
3. All the muscles (mamsa) in the body provide binding and covering to the inner structures and give strength to the body frame. The term mamsa is derived from the root "mam" meaning "to hold firm".
4. The function of adipose tissue (meda) is lubrication (snehana) of the bone joints Meda means "what is oily".
5. The function of bone (asthi) is to support the body. The term asthi is derived from the root "stha" meaning "to stand or to endure".
6. The function of bone marrow and nerve tissue (majja) is to give a

sense of fullness and contentment. It fills the empty spaces in the bones and the cavity inside the skull.

7. The function of the reproductive tissue (shukra) is not only to produce another life, but also to provide strength, energy and stamina. Shukra itself means "seed or luminous". It has two components. 1) a seed element (semen and ovum) and 2) pleasurable fluids released during sexual activity. In men both these components function together, while in women they work separately.

Tissue	Function
Plasma (Rasa)	Provides nutrition to the body
Blood (Rakta)	Gives vital force to the body
Muscle (Mamsa)	Binding, covering
Adipose tissue-fat (Meda)	Lubrication
Bones (Asthi)	Support
Bone Marrow and Nerve tissue (Majja)	Contentment
Reproductive tissue (Shukra)	Reproduction

Waste Products (Mala)

Waste products (mala) are constantly being eliminated from the body. Their physical appearance varies from gaseous and liquid to semi-solid and solid form. Health is maintained when these waste products are eliminated properly. When they accumulate in excess, various diseases are produced.

There are both gross and subtle waste products. The gross waste products (sthoola mala) include urine, feces and sweat. Although they are waste products, they also have to carry out important functions in the body before they are eliminated from the body.

The subtle waste products (sookshma mala) are referred to as Kleda. They are produced in the respective tissue channels. These include exudations eliminated from the epithelial linings of the eyes, nose, ears and genital organs. Additionally, many minute waste products are produced in the body during tissue formation as a result of the digestion of food. These are also considered as subtle waste materials.

WASTE PRODUCT	FUNCTION
Urine (Mutra)	Collects kleda from the different channels for elimination
Feces (Purisha)	a) Provides indirect support to the agni b) gives support and strength to the tissues
Sweat (Sweda)	a) Elimination of kleda through the skin b) retains a part of kleda to provide moisture to the skin

In addition to these gross waste products, each tissue in the body also has a waste, or by product.

TISSUE	WASTE PRODUCT
Plasma (Rasa)	Kapha
Blood (Rakta)	Pitta
Muscle (Mamsa)	ear wax, snot, exudations from the corners of the eyes
Adipose tissue - fat (Meda)	sweat
Bone (Asthi)	hair, nails
Bone marrow and nerve tissue (Majja)	genital secretions - smegma

CHAPTER 5

AYURVEDIC CONSTITUTION - PRAKRUTI

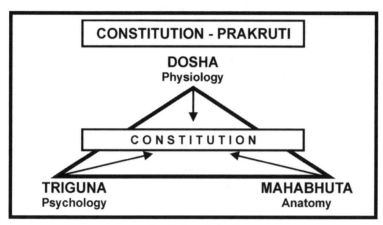

Constitution - Prakruti

Definition of Prakruti

The predominance of elements, gunas, and doshas at the time of conception decides the constitution, or bio-typology of that individual. Once this proportion is set it generally remains permanent for the life span of the individual. Class, family traits, locality, time, age, and individuality also influence the physical constitution

The predominance of the five elements, space, air, fire, water and earth, decides the physical constitution. The predominance of the three gunas, sattva, rajas and tamas, decides the psychological constitution. The predominance of humors (doshas) which are derived from the five elements determines the Doshic Prakruti, which is the functional or energetic condition of the body.

Doshic Functional/Physiological Constitution

With the combination of the three doshas, seven types of constitutions are possible
a) Single dosha predominant- 1) Vata, 2) Pitta, or 3) Kapha,
b) Dual dosha -4) Vata-Pitta, 5) Vata-Kapha, 6) Pitta-Kapha, and
c) Balanced constitution (samaprakruti) with equal proportions of Vata, Pitta and Kapha.

These types are classified by their predominant factor. We find that a purely single Dosha constitution is seldom found, and although a balanced constitution is extremely good, this type is also rare. Many scholars have classified constitution into 10 different types. They include the other three possible combinations, Pitta-Vata, Kapha-Vata and Kapha-Pitta.

In terms of a single dosha predominant constitution, a Vata constitution is usually weaker in terms of resisting disease and thus has a shorter lifespan. Kapha is usually the strongest in terms of disease resistance and enjoys the longest lifespan. Pitta is in between. Samaprakruti, or the constitution in which all three doshas are in equal proportion is considered to be the best in regard to health and longevity. In regard to treatment of the dual constitutions, the Pitta-Kapha type is usually more difficult to treat compared to Vata-Kapha or Vata-Pitta.

Vata Constitution

Those of Vata constitution usually have tall or thin body frames and less strength. Their body weight is low and they have less resistance to disease. Their digestion and metabolism is changeable, hence they cannot form sturdy and stable tissues. Their life span is usually shorter than that of other constitutions. Because of this variable nature in constitution, they cannot perform tasks steadily and continuously. Consequently they may fail in achieving their goals.

Such individuals require a job with little or no strenuous physical activity, in which constant attention is not required, and which is not in a cold or air-conditioned atmosphere. If they are forced to undertake such work they are likely to develop diseases of the nerves and bones, and to suffer from constipation along with loss of weight. When they are balanced they are creative and adaptable.

Pitta Constitution

Those of Pitta constitution have rapid digestive and metabolic activity. They require constant food and drink which is cool in nature. They are usually able to convert food into good quality tissue.

They have soft, oily, and smooth skin. They tend to become bald at an early age, and their hair becomes gray prematurely. They have moderate strength and capacity to work. Although they have a tendency to be hot tempered and become angry easily, they are very intelligent and possess an excellent capacity for comprehension of concepts. They usually possess good knowledge of any subject that interests them and are creative in nature.

Pittas require a job in a cool atmosphere, with some creative activity and intelligent work. They should not deal with chemicals, dyeing material, or petrochemical substances, nor work near heat. They are good leaders and teachers and are usually successful in reaching their goals.

Kapha Constitution

Those of Kapha constitution possess hefty, robust, and thick body frames with good stout musculature. They naturally possess good strength, immunity and vitality, and have a longer life span with good health. They have smooth and deep voices, and are often good looking. The total digestive and metabolic rate in these individuals is very slow and thus they require less food and drink. They are of a calm and quiet nature.

Kapha types can carry out work that is heavy or strenuous. They are also good in maintaining public relations. However they should not work in cold and damp atmospheres. They are have a tendency to gain weight and suffer from joint diseases, heart problems and adult onset diabetes.

Evaluate your Uniqueness - Prakruti

To asses your Prakruti, your natural balance of body humors (doshas), fill out the following form and mark the answer according to your own personal long term nature. If two answers apply for the same question, mark them both. If none is applicable leave it blank. Then tally each column. The column with the most marks is your primary Prakruti. The column with the second largest number is your secondary Prakruti. For example, if you score 18 Vata, 7 Pitta and 4 Kapha, your Prakruti is Vata-Pitta.

VATA	PITTA	KAPHA
PHYSICAL CHRACTERISTICS		
Body frame		
lean, tall or short	medium or short	heavy
Musculature		
thin	smooth, medium	robust, heavy
Skin		
dry, rough	soft, medium, oily	thick, oily

Veins, tendons

exposed, wiry	covered, soft	well hidden

Skin temperature

cold hands and feet	warm	cool

Hair

dry, rough, kinky	soft , thin, fine	thick, oily, wavy

Complexion

dark	pinkish, redish	pale, white

Teeth

irregular	medium, many cavities	even, healthy
dark	yellow	white

Gums

thin, receding	easy to bleed	strong

PHYSIOLOGICAL CHARACTERISTICS

Appetite

variable	strong	low

Thirst

less	always thirsty	less

Bowel movements

often constipated	regular, frequent	regular

Voice

dry, low, cracking	high pitched, sharp	smooth, melodious

Speech

fast, talkative	authoritative	pleasant

Stools

dry, hard, dark	soft, loose	soft, large amount

Urine

less	profuse	normal

Menstruation

painful, irregular   heavy, regular   normal

Sexual drive

variable   strong   moderate

Strength

fair   better   excellent

Exercise tolerance

low   better   good

PSYCHOLOGICAL CHARACTERISTICS

Mental activity

quick, restless   sharp, aggressive   calm, quiet

Thoughts

many, changing   steady, pointed   steady

Concentration

good for short time   better   always good

Sleep

light, interrupted   sound, medium   sound, heavy

Dreams

flying, fearful   aggression   watery, calm

Grasping power

quick   medium   may take longer

Memory

good short term good short and good long term   poor long term

TOTALS

VATA   PITTA   KAPHA

CHAPTER 6

ACTION OF MASSAGE

The word used in many Ayurvedic texts for massage is 'samvahana'. The word mardana has also been used. The term mardana means massage including pressing or rubbing, and also includes other procedures like manipulation of muscles, hairs and joints.

The biological air humor, or Vata dosha, is located in the sense organ of touch (sparshnendriya) which is located in the skin. Of all the sense organs, the sense organ of touch is the most pervading and has an inseparable association with the mind. Thus massage is not only useful for controlling Vata dosha, but also has an effect on the mind.

Massage has been divided into various types. These types include
1. Whole body massage (deha samvahan or deha mardana)
2. Head massage (kesha mardana)
3. Massage to the body with dry powders (udvartana)
4. Massage with herbal paste (utsadana)
5. Reinforced (more pressure) massage with dry powders (udgharshana)
6. Massage with oils (abhyanga)
   (Vatsyayana, Part 1,chapter 3, stanza 15)

Sushruta has mentioned that udvartana, or massage with dry, hot herbal powders, alleviates Vata and Kapha, reduces fat, gives strength to the body and is beneficial to the skin. Utsadana, massage with herbal pastes, is more useful as a cosmetic massage for women. It gives a sense of happiness, makes the skin soft and light and also increases its beauty. Udgharshana, reinforced massage with dry powders, is useful for removing obstructions in the channels. It also removes itching and rashes on the skin. (Su. Chi.24/ 51-43)

The oils and other pastes of herbs, or the medicines applied to the skin for the purpose of massage, penetrate through the skin and reach different tissues and elements of the body. Medicated oil used for massage remains in the skin for 300 seconds (or matras) and then gradually spreads to the blood, muscle, adipose tissue, bone and marrow. The oil takes 100 seconds to penetrate through each of these subsequent tissues according to Sushruta.

Oil massage (abhyanga) is conducive to the healthy growth of the skin. The word 'abhyanga' is derived from the Sanskrit root abhyanj (abhi + anj) which means to anoint or smear. Proper massage with oil removes dirt from the skin, cleans the millions of pores on the skin and helps indirectly in the action of the lungs, large intestine and kidneys. With massage the blood circulation is increased. This helps to accelerate the lymphatic system, which absorbs and eliminates many waste products. The increase in circulation also helps in the exfoliation of superficial dead skin cells. Massage tones the skin and encourages its rejuvenation process. It also helps the skin to maintain its elasticity and strength.

Even if the idea of massage might be attractive, enjoyment of massage is not something that is immediately acceptable to everyone. There are many reasons for this. If you were not handled agreeably as a child, you are unlikely to trust being handled as an adult. Fortunately the body is designed in such a way as to be constantly massaging itself, and this can give us some confidence to being with a masseur. The diaphragm muscles between the chest and abdomen alternatively compress and release the digestive organs with each deep breath. Even the slightest movement of the limb muscles puts pressure on the nearby veins to keep peripheral circulation flowing. The arms, allowed to swing by our sides as we walk, relax the muscles of the back. If we are able to imagine this, we are on the way to appreciating the advantages offered by applied massage. In order to gain full benefit we need to be totally passive and surrender to the touch of a skilled masseur or therapist.

There is a great deal of scientific evidence that the state of the mind and the nervous system is reflected in the state of the musculature. A relaxed person tends to have relaxed muscles, while a tense person has tense muscles along with aches and pains. Using massage or body work to relax the muscles is one route into the subconscious and provides relaxation to the mind. Additionally, nerve endings can be stimulated or soothed depending on the depth of the massage and the various types of movements used by the masseur.

Human beings need to touch and be touched. Animal and human research shows that individuals deprived of physical contact are insecure, poorly adjusted and more prone to illness. Massage is a very sensitive and sensitizing form of human contact, whose medium is touch, a sense to which animals as well as human being's are especially responsive. The first experience of massage is obtained when the fetus is delivered from the uterus due to rhythmic contractions of the uterine muscles. After we are born, holding, rocking, washing and caressing by the parent prepares our body for its independence. Animals also are aware of the action of massage on their newborn. Many animals lick the entire body of the newborn immediately after the birth. This helps not only to clean their body but gives them a soothing massage with the tongue.

Massage increases the circulation of the blood and lymph. It has been shown by various scientific experiments that more blood flows through the tissues during and after the friction or rubbing of massage. Experiments have also shown that there is an increase in the number of red blood cells along with an increase in the flow of lymph. During massage, waste products such as lactic acid and congested blood in the exhausted muscles are removed and the muscles become refreshed. Massage also improves the local and general nutrition of the body.

CHAPTER 7

BASIC STROKES OF MASSAGE

Massage Techniques

Massage is not just rubbing or pressing on the body or application of oil. To receive the full benefit from massage, one needs to understand the systematic way of performing massage. The following strokes of massage were formulated by Swedish Professor Henry King in the 19th century

Friction or Effleurage (Gharshana)

Friction massage is also known as Effleurage. This is a "connective tissue massage". This can be done by using the thumbs, fingertips, knuckles or palm of the hand. This is very useful for improving blood circulation in the body. In friction massage, more pressure is applied on muscular part while gentle pressure is given on the bony parts. The following are sub-types of friction massage.

a) Towards the heart (pratiloma) - This should be done on the arms and legs by using pressure of the thumb or palm of the hand. This is useful for treating varicose veins.

b) Away from the heart (anuloma) - This type of massage is used during whole body massage.

c) Circular - Mainly for the big muscles on the arms and legs. The patients hand or leg is held with one hand while the other hand performs circular pressure. Carry out this technique from the hand to the shoulder or from the sole of the foot to the hip joint.

d) Zig-Zag - On the spinal cord or sternum, lower to upper, using fingers or the palm of the hand.

e) Round - Useful for flat surfaces or joints for Vata-Pitta or Kapha type people.

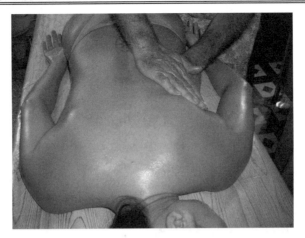

Back Massage - Round Movements

Kneading (Peedana)

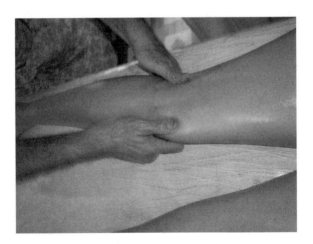

Kneading with Thumbs

a) Superficial kneading (avapeedana). Also referred to as pinching. Using the thumb and index finger, the skin is lifted and gently pinched. This is useful for improving the peripheral or capillary circulation. It can be given in any direction. But it is different from lymphatic massage. This is useful in skin diseases.

b) Deep kneading (pra-peedana). Deep kneading can be divided into several types as follows.

Petrissage - By using the palms and giving parallel deep pressure to parts of the body. This method is mainly useful for the muscular parts of the hands and legs to improve deep and superficial circulation.

Palmer kneading - Using the palms over the abdomen, back and chest.

Fist kneading - Used mainly on the abdomen. This method is useful for relieving chronic constipation.

Fist Massage on Abdomen

Digital kneading (anguli peedana) - Using the fingers to knead deeply. Useful for the back, face, etc.

Rounding

This is a very fast movement using both hands. The objective is to move the muscles in a round direction.

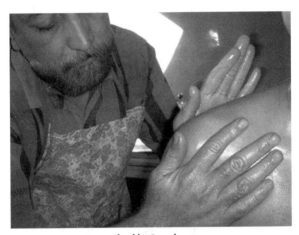

Shoulder Rounding

Wringing or Twisting (Udveshtana)

The muscles are twisted by using both hands. In this type of massage, rolling and twisting actions are carried out.

Chucking

Lifting the muscle upwards slightly, holding, then releasing. It is used mainly for sprains and catching types of pain. Sprains are when the ligaments connecting the joints are overstretched or torn. Catching types of pain are produced due to tender muscles.

Stroking (Trasana)

Fingers and palms are used for this method by giving more or less pressure. This is useful for the head, back, chest and abdomen. There are several kinds of stokes.
a) Digital stroking - Very gentle massage to stimulate bony parts or bony prominences like the forehead, tibia and vertebral column. This should preferably be done using the tips of the fingers.
b) Palmer stroking - Palms of both hands should be used on the borders of the muscles of the thighs, calfs and buttocks.

c) Knuckle Stroking - Using the knuckles, this stroke is given mainly where thick muscles are located such as on the chest and back.
d) Reflex stroking - Using a particular type of instrument to strike the muscle, such as when a small rubber hammer is used to produce a knee jerk reaction. This is very helpful for improving reflexes in diseases related to Vata, and also improves the activity of the nerves.

Percussion (Praharana)

In this type the muscles or the body part is stroked by using the fingers or the palms of both hands. It is very useful for improving metabolism and local temperature of the body part. In Vata and Pitta types it is useful in removing obstructions in the channels to allow the free flow of the doshas. The following types of percussion are used.
a) Digital (vadana)- Using the tips of the fingers, gentle strokes are given. This is useful for head and chest massage.
b) Using the palm of the hand (aasphalana or tadana). Useful for all over the body.
c) Hand cupping (samputaka). The hand is formed into a cup and used to tap the body part up and down. This makes a slight suction and the skin is lifted with each tap. It is useful on muscular parts of the body.
d) Pounding. Done with the fists it is useful for heavy and strong muscles. It improves the temperature and circulation of that part of the muscle or the body.

Vibrations (Kampa or Harshana)

The vibrations produced by massage are useful for activating both superficial and deep movement of the part. In this method the masseur vibrates his own hand and produces vibrations to the part of the body by using the fingers and the palm. This method improves circulation of the part and removes obstructions in the channels. After friction massage, vibrations are given to clean the channels. Tingling sensations, numbness, heaviness of the part, partial loss of muscles and atrophy is treated by superficial and deep vibrations and movement of the body part.

Joint movements (Sandhi Chalana)

In this type of massage the joints are moved and are also massaged. In daily life we observe that most people do not carry out any exercise. Hence, movements of certain joints are restricted and ultimately become stiff. Massage with gradual increase in joint movements improves flexibility, removes congestion and helps free movements of the joints. Please note that in cases of frozen shoulder and tennis elbow this type of massage is associated with medicated fomentation (moist heat).
Multiple movements are possible in hip and shoulder joints such as

flexion, extension, abduction, adduction and circumlocution. Flexion, extension & rotary movements are possible in ankle and wrist joints, while flexion and extension are possible in elbow and knee joints.

Touch (Sparsha)

After completing all the above types of massage, the patient needs a gentle touch for a soothing effect. This can be done all over the body or a part of the body to conclude the massage, using a very gentle touch with the hands.

Gentle Friction Massage (Mardana)

Friction massage (mardana) is usually done after abhyanga (heavy application of oil). In this method, a gentle massage is used with fingers, thumbs and palms. Skill is more important than power. Patting, gentle rubbing, soft squeezing and vibrations are used. Movements are mainly to be performed according to the shape of the muscles.

CHAPTER 8

AYURVEDIC MASSAGE

In the previous chapter on the history of massage we have seen that many countries and cultures have a tradition of massage. In this context, often the question is asked "What is special about Ayurvedic massage ?". Ayurvedic massage has a long history as a part of Ayurvedic treatment. It is unique in the sense that it considers the principles of the five basic elements, the biological humors or energies, the concept of agni, as well as the formation of toxins (ama).

The aim of Ayurveda is to balance the energies inside the body for optimum health To achieve this balance, the study of the fundamental concept of Prakruti, your constitutional uniqueness, is essential. Prakruti not only determines which massage oils or direction the massage should be given, it also helps to determine the best diet, lifestyle, occupation, climate and other factors which allow you to be aa healthy as possible.

Ayurvedic massage uses a variety of substances such as simple oils, medicated oils, flours of foods like lentils or chic peas for dry massage, aromatic oils, powders of various herbs, milk, wooden rollers, and rough gloves made of cotton cloth or silk. There are also different types of massage which vary according to the need of the patient and the disease he is suffering from. Various supplementary procedures like swedana (sweating therapy), nasya (administration of substances through the nose), shiro basti (retaining oil in a open cap on the head) and shirodhara (running a stream of oil onto the forehead) can be given along with Ayurvedic massage to enhance the effects. Ayurvedic massage also plays a very important role in the rejuvenation of the body, called Rasayana, for achieving longevity.

Timing of massage

Massage should preferably be done in the early morning hours, when the stomach of the patient is empty. It can also be done 3 to 4 hours after eating. It should not be done immediately after taking food.

Requirements for Massage

The room for the massage should be warm and comfortable. Massage can be done either on a massage table, which is about the height of ones waist, or it can be done on the floor. The table should be properly covered with a clean white cloth so that the patient is comfortable during the massage procedure. In procedures such as taila dhara (oil drip on the head) a special type of wooden table called a droni should be used which allows for the recovery of the massage oil from the body of the patient. The masseur should be healthy, not suffering from any contagious skin disease and should trim their nails so that during the massage they will not harm the patient.

Abhyanga

Abhyanga means the application of plain or medicated oil to the body. The oil should be according to ones constitution, age, season, particular disease and the atmosphere. For massage, a detailed anatomical knowledge of muscles (peshi), joints (sandhi), and vital areas (marma) is essential.

Types of Abhyanga

1) Oil massage in health.
2) Oil massage in different diseases.
3) Whole body massage.
4) Massage to a part of the body.
5) Self (Auto) massage.
6) Synchronized massage.

Benefits of Abhyanga

1) Beneficial to the eyes (Drushti Prasad Kara) - Proper massage around the eyes and face makes the eyes beautiful and shining. It increases the acuity of vision and helps to prevent blindness and diseases of the eyes. For treating disorders like myopia, massage to the scalp and soles of the feet is very useful. Massage to the kurcha and kurchashira marmas, located on the hands and feet, is always beneficial for the eyes.

2) Nourishes the body (Pushtikara) - Massage makes the muscles strong, increases stamina, vitality and virility. It also helps for elimination of waste products like sweat, urine and feces.

3) Promotes Longevity (Ayu Kara) - The functions of the vital organs and tissues can be improved and the life span can be increased through the practice of regular massage therapy.

4) Induces proper sleep (Swapna Kara) - Physical and mental feelings of well being, nourishment, strength, increased sexual ability and the ability to perceive knowledge depend upon proper sleep. Massage is a powerful agent which induces sound sleep.

5) Makes the skin soft and silky (Sutwak Kara) - Massage improves the skin complexion and makes it lustrous and beautiful. It also resists premature wrinkles, unwanted hair and warts, and increases immunity against skin diseases.

6) Makes the skin firm (Dardhya Kara)- By properly removing waste products and providing nutrition, massage promotes sturdiness and firmness of the skin.

7) Increases strength of the skin (Klesha Sahatwa) - Massage increases the resisting power against physical and mental pressure, stress and strain, agonies, sorrows and anxiety. Massage also improves our general tolerance and patience.

8) Increases immunity of the skin (Abhighata Sahatwa) - Massage induces speedy recovery of wounds and fractures and also resists permanent debility or deformity after fractures and accidents.

9) Removes fatigue (Shrama Hara) - Massage overcomes fatigue. Fatigue due to routine work, mental stress and strain can be corrected by regular massage.

10) Regulates Vata - Prevents and corrects disorders caused by Vata. Vata regulates all the sensory and motor functions of the nervous system, along with regulating the activities of Pitta and Kapha. Thus, Vata plays a critical role in the creation, sustenance and decay of the body. Therefore, for an individual to be healthy and happy, Vata must always be kept in equilibrium. The two sense organs associated with Vata are hearing and touch, via the skin. Skin is the main sensory organ through which, with the help of massage, Vata can be kept in equilibrium.

Massage should be done regularly. As a person must take food daily, so also should they resort to massage daily. For a normal, healthy person massage should be done before they take a bath. Massage is very helpful before performing physical exercise and is also useful for those who practice yoga. Massage should only be performed after the patient has digested the food from the previous meal.

In short, the secret of youth and beauty is the proper circulation of the vital life fluids and the regular discharge of waste materials. In this regard massage plays a very important role. Massage helps keep you feeling young, vital, beautiful and healthy. The body can be compared to tree. If the roots of the tree are given water regularly, it will live and be healthy for a long time. Similarly, if the body of an individual is oiled properly through massage, they will live a long life without any decay or disease.

Therapeutic Indications of Abhyanga

1) For general weakness - Massage should preferably be given every day to remove wear and tear of the tissues, relief from fatigue, to give strength to the muscles and growth of the body. It is indicated from childhood to old age.

2) Disorders of the joints - All types of arthritis, i.e. osteo-arthritis (asthi gata vata), rheumatoid arthritis (sandhigata vata), rheumatic arthritis

(amavata), spondilytis, disorders of the vertebral column and gout (va tarakta).

3) Diseases of the muscles such as myositis (muscle inflammation with pain), spasm, atrophy, various types of myopathies, etc.

4) Nervous system disorders - Neuralgia (pain due to inflammation in the nerves), sciatica, poliomyelitis, hemiplegia, paraplegia and cerebral palsy.

5) Drug addiction - As a preventive and therapeutic in withdrawal syn drome.

6) Feminine problems - Dysmenorrhea (painful menstruation), oligom enorrhea (sparse or infrequent menstruation), menorrhagia (excessive flow during menstruation), leukorrhea (an abnormally large amount of white or yellow discharge of mucus from the vagina) and menopaus al syndrome.

7) Circulatory problems - After myocardial infarction, ischaemic heart dis ease, functional heart disease, cold hands and feet due to bad circula tion and varicose veins.

8) Sports diseases - Tennis elbow, lumbago, frozen shoulder, shoulder and backache, sprains, strains and aches, etc.

9) Psychological problems - Schizophrenia, illusions, depression, negative thinking, constant worry, loss of memory and insomnia.

10) Metabolic disorders - Obesity, loss of weight and stamina, increase of the digestive and tissue fires.

11) Post delivery - Massage after delivery to both the mother and child is done to relieve the Vata vitiation (increase) in mothers and to enhance the immunity in children.

Contraindications for Abhyanga

Patients suffering from fever, high ama (toxins), skin inflammations, indigestion, those who have skin which is sensitive to inflammation or whom Panchakarma (Ayurvedic cleansing procedures) has been given.

Abhyanga in Therapy

Before therapeutic abhyanga, the physician or the masseur must examine the patient thoroughly to determine his constitution, type of disease, vitiated (abnormal) dosha and the presence of ama (toxins). The following form should be properly filled out.

Examination of the patient

Name, age, sex, address.
History of chief complaints and their duration.
Personal health history.
Family health history.

General examination. This should include examination of the tongue, urine, feces and pulse to determine whether the patient has a large amount of toxins (ama) in the body. The presence of toxins (ama) can be determined by noting if there is a heavy coating on the tongue which can not be removed by scraping the tongue with a tongue scraper or small spoon. Additionally, if the urine is turbid (cloudy) with a foul smell and the feces are foul smelling and sink instead of floating in water, this also indicates that toxins (ama) are present in the body.

If the patient has a large amount of toxins (ama) in the body, massage should not be given.

Later on a systemic examination should be done to find out the type of disease and the type of vitiated (abnormal) dosha. Oil for massage can be selected according to these findings.

General Procedure for Massage
Requirements
Massage table, vessel containing oil, hot water bath.

Main Procedure
Usually this is done in seven positions as follows -
1) With the patient in a sitting position, apply a cooling type of oil to the head, and massage the head properly. Give attention to the marmas (vital areas) such as adhipati, seemanta and the other marmas in the region of the head. Using the proper massage oil, apply oil to the ears, face, palms and soles of the feet. Continue by applying oil to the neck then downwards to the chest and back.
2) Ask the patient to lie on their back.
Foot Massage - Depending on whether the patient is lying on a table or on the floor, the masseur should sit or stand at the side of the patient. Apply plenty of oil to the sole of the foot after cleaning the same with a towel. Next use a brisk, friction (gharshana) type massage on the sole of the foot, massaging the dorsum of the foot. Stretch the toes of the foot and massage them also.
Leg massage - Apply oil from the ankle to the knee joint. Give friction massage to the calf muscles. Apply oil from the knee to the groin,coming down with three or four rotary sweeps and with occasional strokes with the front and back of the fingers. Carry out a twisting, soothing and vibratory massage to the entire leg. The masseur should then raise the leg of the patient and keep it on their own shoulder, rubbing from the foot to the hip with both hands at least six

times. The masseur should then put the leg down and flex the leg a the knee. Give a circular massage to the ankle and knee joints.

Thigh massage - All the thigh muscles are big. They require kneading using the fingers Later a pounding massage by fists also.

Massage to abdomen - The movement of massage on the abdomen should be circular and it should be light. Proper attention should be given to the important marmas like hridaya, nabhi and basti.

Massage to the chest- Apply a large amount of oil on the front portion of the chest Start massaging at the level of the last rib on each side and proceed upwards and inwards and then outwards and upwards. Then start from the midline of the chest and massage both the arms up to the middle and back to the chest.

In the case of females, give a circular massage to the breast. As far as possible do not touch the nipples during the massage. Massage the breasts from the periphery to the center.

3) Ask the patient to take the left lateral position.

In this position, massage can be done to the right flank and right hand and foot.

4) Ask the patient to lie on their back.

Hand massage - It should start from the nails if the massage is being done for cosmetic purposes. Put a drop of oil at the nail bed and massage. Apply oil to the palm and start massaging the front and back portion of the palm. Apply a circular massage to the fingers and their joints. Stretch the fingers slightly.

Arm massage- Apply oil to the whole arm from the wrist to the shoulder joint. Give a circular massage to the wrist, elbow and shoulder joints. Follow with a rolling type of massage to the entire arm.

5) The patient should then take the right lateral position.

In this position, massage can be done to the region of the left flank and left hand and foot.

6. Again ask the patient to lie on their back and massage the chest, abdomen and both the extremities.

7) Lastly, ask the patient to assume a sitting position and massage all the body once again in this position.

Massage to the back - Unless it has been specifically indicated, the patient is usually not asked to lie on the abdomen to avoid excessive pressure on the abdominal organs. Massage to the back should be done in a sitting, left and right lateral position.

An exception to the general rule of not having the patient lie on the abdomen is in the Kerala type of massage. In a Kerala type massage the massage is started with the patient lying on their abdomen, and they are then given massage from the legs up to the head. The above steps, 1 through 7, are then performed.

Neck Massage - Start massaging the vertebrae from the cervical region. Move down slowly to the thoracic region, then to the lumbar region. Massage each vertebra with special attention to its ligaments and the muscles attached to it.

Post procedure

After the massage the patient can be given fomentation if it has been prescribed. Otherwise, remove the excess oil by using dry powders or with the help of a towel. Application of dry powders of vacha (calamus) or other powders of lentils like chickpea is useful in removing excess oil from the skin. The patient is then asked to take a warm bath or shower and is allowed to rest.

Massage According to Constitution

The direction, rate, oil and amount of pressure varies depending on the constitution and current balance, or imbalance of the patient.

Massage for Vata Constitution

Vata type people are dry and cool by nature. To balance the dryness, larger amounts of oil are used. To balance the coolness, warming oils, which have been heated, are preferred. Sesame oil is best for reducing Vata. It removes dryness, coldness, stiffness and pain, lubricates dry skin and protects the joints.

Medicated oils such as dashamula oil, which is a preparation made from ten different roots, or oil prepared from the group of herbs included in Jeevaniya or Brimhaniya, are the best for Vata. Similarly ashwagandha (withania somnifera), bala (sida cordifolia), narayana or mahanarayana oil, which includes shatavari (Aaparagus racemosus) along with 23 other herbs and milk, can also be used.

Essential oils such as ginger, basil, camphor and eucalyptus, which have a hot potency are typically used. Vata types are very sensitive to touch, so a gentle massage with warm oil should be given. Massage should be done daily, in the early morning, or before a warm bath in the evening. Massage strokes are given in the direction of away from the heart.

Massage for Pitta Constitution

Pitta types have a rapid metabolism and a tendency toward fever and inflammatory diseases. Their skin is sensitive and easily gets rashes or inflammations. Cooling massage oils should be used. Coconut or sandalwood oil is best. Both these oils calm the mind and cool the body. Sunflower oil is also useful for inflamed skin. Medicated oils can be prepared from cardamom (ela), jatamansi, myristica fragrans, musta, chandana, nagakeshara and karpura. Essential oils such as lemongrass, lavender, jasmine and sandalwood are also useful. (See Pitta massage oils in Chapter 14) Massage for Pitta should be of a medium pressure, with the strokes alternating away from and then towards the heart.

Massage for Kapha Constitution

Kapha types have thick and oily skin and need massage to improve their circulation and lymph drainage. The best massage for these people is with powders of herbs with a dry and hot potency. Oil should be used sparingly and should be of a hot potency such as mustard or sesame. Powders of herbs such as calamus (vacha), dry ginger or dashamula and the powders of various lentils like chick pea or bengal gram are typically used. Medicated oil can be prepared with bilwa, dashamula, guggulu, shilajita, devadaru and tagara. Essential oils such as basil, ginger, clove or eucalyptus can be used. (See Kapha massage oil in Chapter 14) The massage should be vigorous and deep with strokes towards the heart.

Constitution (dosha)	Amount of oil
Vata	100 ml
Pitta	60 ml
Kapha	10 ml

The rate, direction and pressure that should be used vary depending on the patients constitution or imbalance. The following rules are applied for friction type massage.

For Vata disorders and constitutions -

The massage should be away from the heart (anuloma).

For Pitta disorders and constitutions -

Combinations of anuloma and pratiloma should be used. The massage stroke is away from the heart, then reversed back towards the heart, then repeated.

For Kapha disorders and constitutions -

Pratiloma should be used (towards the heart).

Direction of Massage	Pressure	Rate	Oil
Vata - away from the heart (anuloma)	gentle	up to 30 strokes per minute	Sesame oil
Pitta - (anuloma and pratiloma)	moderate	40 strokes per minute	Coconut or sunflower oil
Kapha - towards the heart (pratiloma)	deep	50 to 60 strokes per minute	Dry powders of calamus or red lentils with a small amount of olive or mustard oil

Dual Dosha Constitution

In the case of a healthy patient with a dual constitution, the direction of massage should be according to the predominant dosha. Therefore, for a Pitta-Vata constitution where Pitta is predominant, the direction of massage would alternate away, then towards the heart.

Vata/Pitta- Use less oil than a pure Vata. Olive, coconut or sunflower oil should be used. The direction of massage should be away from the heart (anuloma).

Pitta/Kapha - Use sunflower or coconut oil along with dry powders of legumes. The direction of massage should be away from the heart (anuloma).

Vata/Kapha - Since this is a Vata/Kapha constitution we use a small amount of oil along with a large amount of powder. Using dry powders alone would aggravate Vata as Vata naturally has a dry quality. Using oil alone would aggravate Kapha due to the naturally oily quality of Kapha. Use dry powders of various hot herbs such as calamus (vacha - acorus calamus), or dry powders of lentils and legumes such as chic pea. The oil can be sesame or a hot and penetrating oil such as mustard or medicated calamus. First apply the oil then apply the powder. The direction of massage should be away from the heart (anuloma).

Direction of Massage For Dual Dosha Disorders

In a diseased patient with more than one dosha out of balance, the direction of massage should be according to the dosha which is most aggravated.

Udvartana

Udvartana means massage with pressure. There are two types of Udvartana.

1) Dry - With herbal powders (recommended in obesity).

2) Unctuous - Application of oil or oily herbal pastes (useful in debility).

Benefits

1. Removes foul smell from the body.
2. Cures heaviness, drowsiness, itching and diseases caused by accumulation of waste products, excessive sweating and disfiguration of the skin.
3. Alleviates Vata.
4. Helps in mobilization of excess Kapha and fat.
5. Produces stability of the limbs.
6. Promotes skin texture.
7. Improves the circulation in the channels.
8. Stimulates various doshas responsible for metabolic process in the skin and keeps the skin healthy.
9. Especially promotes the complexion of the skin and also helps in removing unwanted hair from the face and body.

Udgharshana

In this method dry powders of medicinal plants are used and the massage is done by applying reinforced friction.

This type of massage has the following benefits.

1. It cures itching, urticaria and diseases caused by Vata.
2. It produces stability and lightness in the body.
3. It promotes the activities of bhrajaka Pitta in the skin and helps in removing sweat from the openings of the sweat glands.

For Vata disorders and constitutions

Powders of amalaki (emblica officinalis), vacha (acorus calamus) and triphala are advised.

For Pitta disorders and constitutions

Powders of sandalwood, shatavari (asparagus racemosus), sariva (indian sarsaparila), musta (Cyperus rotundus), usheera (vetivera) and anantamula (Hemidesmus indicus) are beneficial.

For Kapha disorders and constitution

Use powders of haritaki, vacha (acorus calamus), nimba (azadirachata indica), and arjuna (terminalia arjuna). Mustard seed powder and powder of red lentils can be used in small amounts.

Both Udvartana and Udgharshana types of massage should preferably be done after abhyanga and Mardana and before taking a bath.

Self Massage

Self massage, also called auto massage, should be done daily by every individual to maintain health. Every person should use oil that is suitable according to their own constitution as explained above. There is a saying in the Kerala region of India that a person should use a small amount of money on massage oils rather than giving a large amount of money to the doctor for curing diseases. This supports the idea that daily oil massage, abhyanga, can prevent various diseases.

Requirements

Massage oil, Hair oil, Hot water bath, Cleansing powder.

Procedure

Usually different oils are used for the head than for the rest of the body. Oils which are cool in potency should be used on the head. An exception to this general rule of using cooling oils on the head would be in the case of treating diseases using a warming oil, such as mustard oil, on a particular area on the head. (see Marma massage in chapter 10)

Almost all oils, since they are oily, heavy and warm, act as anti-Vata. Sesame oil is the best oil for Vata constitution, and if properly processed has anti-oxidant qualities. To process sesame oil, heat it to about 110 degrees, then let the oil cool before storing. When you are ready for massage, warm the required oil in a water bath to 39 degrees Celsius/102 degrees F. Sit on a stool or chair in a warm bathroom or other comfortable place. Pour the warm oil in your palm so that you can check the temperature of the oil before applying.

1. First apply oil to the top of the head and massage the head for one minute. When massaging the scalp use the fingertips first to give stimulation to the scalp area and then one can use the palm for general application of oils to the head. Next massage the face, front and back of the neck, and head with the palms. Give special attention to the head marmas such as adhipati (at the highest point on the head), seemanta (along the joints of the skull) and shankha (at a point halfway between the outside corner of the eye and the tragus of the ear. The tragus is the flap of skin which covers the opening of the ear.

2. Next, using an oil which is suitable for body massage, massage the external ear by holding the right ear lobe with the thumb and index finger. Use the tip of the index finger to massage the innermost part of the ear. Do the massage in the same manner to the left ear also.

3. Begin massaging the arms with back and forth movements. Use circular movements over the joints.
4. Apply oil to the chest and abdomen. Pour a little oil in the nabhi marma, located at the umbilicus area. On the abdomen, gentle circular movements should be used. Use gentle massage to the nabhi, basti and hridaya marmas.
5. Next apply oil to the soles of the feet and legs followed by massage. It is best to leave the oil on the body at least 15 to 30 minutes. Use cleansing powders of calamus (vacha) or lentil flour to remove any excess oil from the skin depending on the constitution or imbalance. A small amount of oil should be left on the skin. Follow with a warm bath or shower.

Synchronized massage

This is performed by two masseurs in simultaneous and synchronized movements. The advantage of this type of massage is that both sides of the patient is massaged at the same time. This gives maximum comfort and relaxation to the patient. It is important in this massage that both masseurs exert the same amount and type of pressure while massaging. They must have worked together for a long time to achieve the proper effect of synchronized movements.

Massage for Pregnant Women

For pregnant women, massage should be given very carefully and it should be for as long as the women desires. If regular massage is given to a pregnant women it ensures a painless delivery.

If the patient is lying down, give her plenty of support with the help of cushions under her neck, back and at any other position she needs to feel comfortable. For abdominal massage use light strokes. Apply sufficient oil around the abdomen and carry out a soothing circular type of massage.

To help the nipple develop properly for breast feeding, and to allow for the proper flow of breast milk, a female masseur should perform a breast massage. By performing breast massage the channels which carry breast milk (stanyavaha srotas) are stimulated and any blockages are removed. Breast massage also helps to avoid cracking of the nipple. The breast massage should be done from the outer portion of the breast, moving in towards the nipple, using both hands.

For problems like backache, massage should be given to the back and at the lumbar region with the patient in a sitting position. Very gentle strokes and pressure is applied to the entire vertebral column and back to relieve stiffness.

Massage to the legs also should be done which will relieve the problems of swelling of the legs and varicose veins. Before labor, and after delivery, women have some common complaints of morning sickness, heartburn, sore breasts, constipation, sleep problems, stretch marks etc. In such cases choose a correct oil according to the constitution and give a very gentle massage. This should be complemented with a good diet and plenty of rest.

Massage after delivery (Mother massage)

During labor it is very helpful to give a back massage. Immediately after delivery there is Vata vitiation in the mother, as she looses a lot of energy along with plasma and blood. There is much physical and mental strain on the body during the process of delivery. There is pain before and after the delivery due to the contraction of the muscles of the uterus and other muscles in the area of back.

Massage helps the system to reorganize itself and also gives relief to the mother. The child remains in the womb of the mother for a period of nine months and during this time the musculature in the abdominal region becomes stretched. After delivery, therefore, there are stretch marks on the skin of the abdomen known as stria gravidum. Regular massage after delivery helps to remove these stretch marks and gives strength to the abdominal muscles which can prevent hernias in this region. Three months of massage will help the body to acquire the same shape as before pregnancy. The massage is done in the same style as that of abhyanga and is preferably given in the seven positions explained earlier.

Baby Massage

Massage to a new born baby is an old tradition of Ayurveda. The baby massage begins after the umbilical cord becomes dry and falls off, 8 to 15 days after birth.

Requirements

Warm room, warm water bath, vessel containing oil, dry powder of calamus.

Benefits of baby massage

1. Stimulates circulation.
2. Gives good passive exercise.
3. Stimulates digestion.
4. Boosts immunity.
5. Controls Vata dosha - The skin is the biggest organ of our body and proper massage by oils or medicated powders keeps Vata dosha in control. It was previously thought that oil applied to the skin does not get absorbed in the body. It is now known that not only does it get ab-

sorbed, but it also stimulates various internal physiological functions.

6. Maintains and regulates body temperature. It also improves resistance power.

Procedure

A newborn baby instinctively responds to touch and massage. A women masseur who knows this traditional massage usually performs the baby massage.

Position of the masseur -

The women masseur usually sits on the ground with her legs stretched out in front and joined together. She then takes the baby on her lap and starts pouring warm oil on the anterior fontanel. In the newborn this point is very delicate, as the bones of the skull have not yet fused together. Very gentle massage should be done with ample oil placed in the hollow space at this point.

Next the baby should be put on their back and given light strokes down to the chest and abdomen, gently stroking both the hands and legs. Massage is then given to the foot, slightly stretching the toes and rubbing the feet, followed by massage to the soles of the feet.

Keep the baby on the abdomen, face down, and massage the legs, back and hands as well. 30 days after birth medium pressure massage can be applied to the child. Squeeze both the hands and the legs and give passive exercise to both extremities. For the back give gentle pounding and pressure using an open palm. Finish the massage by giving soothing strokes.

Post procedure

After the massage give the baby a warm bath. To remove any excess oil, apply powder of bengal gram or any other dry powder of lentils which are available. After the bath quickly dry the body and apply powder of calamus on the head at the Adhipati marma (see chapter 10). Calamus is hot in potency and dry in quality. This prevents vitiation (increase) of Kapha thereby avoiding colds and cough. Wrap the baby tightly in cotton cloth and allow them to sleep peacefully.

For baby massage the best medicated oils are

1. Bala oil - Bala (sida cordifolia) in Sanskrit means child. This herb is extremely useful in all disorders of children. The oil is prepared using bala juice, bala paste (kalka), sesame oil and cow's milk.
2. Chandan-bala-lakshadi oil.
3. Narayan oil.
4. Baby massage oil (see chapter 14).

CHAPTER 9

KERALA MASSAGE

Massage has been developed extensively in the Kerala region of India. Kerala massage was originally developed to give relief from fatigue to the performers of the lengthy Kathakali dances. These dances usually begin at 9:00 pm and continue until 4:00 am. The following are some of the specialized Kerala massage techniques.

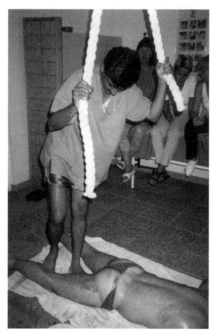

Chavitti

Chavitti

Chavitti means feet. Compared to massage by the hands, the feet can put a lot of pressure on the patient's body. This method is used to give a deep massage It is more useful for robust Kapha type constitution people, as well as for fitness and flexibility for dancers and athletes.

Preliminary procedure

First the patient is given a whole body, abhyanga massage, with suitable oil according to his constitution.

Main procedure

A heavy rope is hung horizontally at a height of about 6 to7 feet, depending on the height of the masseur. Alternately, two ropes can be hung vertically, or instead of rope, the masseur can use rings attached to the ceiling. The patient is then asked to lie on the floor on a carpet. A flat pan which is filled with a suitable warm oil is kept alongside the patient. The masseur takes hold of the rope, dips his foot in the oil and carries out a massage using the feet. Like the other types of massage, this massage is given for 30 to 45 minutes. Charaka has explained this procedure as padaghata.

Post procedure

After the massage, the patient is asked to take a warm bath and rest at least for 30 minutes. He should avoid exposure to cold wind and should refrain from taking cold foods and drinks for the day.

Pizhichil

Pizhi means squeezing and chil means vigorous synchronized movements of massage. This technique is a combination of oleation (oiling) and sudation (heating) therapy. Normally during oil massage the oil is warmed to body temperature. In pizhichil the oil is warmed to about 102 degrees which gives a heating effect to the procedure

Requirements

In this type of massage the oil which has been warmed to the proper temperature is put into a pan. Eight to ten cotton cloth pieces are soaked in the warm oil then squeezed allowing the oil to run over the affected part of the body.

Main procedure

The patient is asked to lie on a wooden droni. This is a special table prepared for this purpose. The table is designed to quickly collect the used oil from the massage, which then is reheated and used again during the procedure. As usual, first gentle massage is given. This procedure is carried out with four masseurs who massage the patient with synchronize movements. About 1 liter of oil is used for massage.

Post procedure

After 30 to 45 minutes, the oil on the body of the patient is removed by applying flour of lentils followed by massage for 5 minutes. A light layer of oil is then reapplied, followed by a warm bath or shower, then rest. This type of massage is excellent for alleviating Vata disorders. It also tones up the body and reduces fatigue.

Uzhichil

This is a type of abhyanga in which special oils are prepared according to the Kerala tradition. Dhanvatara oil, kottamchukadi oil, chandan bala lakshadi oil and sahacharadi oil are some of the important oils used in Kerala massage. The requirements and other procedures are the same as that of Pizhichil.

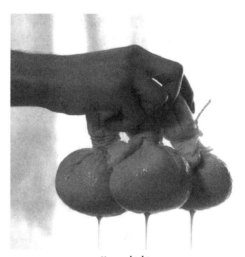

Navarakizhi

Navarakizhi
or
Shashti Shalika Pinda Sweda

Requirements

Massage table or wooden droni, cows milk - 1 liter, decoction of bala (Sida cordifolia) - 1 liter, navara rice - 180 grams.

Navara is a special type of rice which grows to maturity in 60 days. Some traditions first cook the rice in milk while others prefer to cook the rice first in water then put the rice into the boiled milk and the decoction. The cooked rice is then divided into six equal parts and each one is put into a piece of cloth. The corners are gathered to form a ball and tied with thread, leaving a tuft of cloth which is used as a handle. This ball is referred to as a bolus.

Main Procedure

All the boluses are kept in a vessel containing the bala decoction and this vessel is then heated. The patient is given abhyanga with suitable medicated oil. Next, two masseurs begin massaging the patient with the bolus. When the bolus becomes cool it should be replaced by a warm one. This relay of warm boluses with cool ones should be done continuously until the bala decoction is gone. This massage with the warm bolus should be done in all seven positions as explained earlier under abhyanga.

Post procedure

After the massage, the paste of rice is removed from the boluses and is massaged on the body of the patient for five minutes. The paste is then gently wiped from the body. Once again a light coating of oil should be applied, the patient should take a warm bath or shower, then be allowed to rest.

Precaution

The masseur should check, on his own hand, the temperature of the bolus before applying it to the patient.

This treatment can be carried out on alternate days for from 7 to 14 days.

Indications -

Diseases of Vata, nervous system disorders, rheumatism, arthritis, muscular dystrophy, muscular weakness, paresis, paralysis and for general health.

Contra indications -

Excessive Kapha diseases, obesity, asthma and high fever.

Kizhi

Kizhi means poultice. Different poultices with various herbs are prepared according to the specific disorder such as nervous, muscular or orthopedic complaints. The massage is performed with these poultices. This is also known as Elakizhi.

CHAPTER 10

MARMA MASSAGE

Marma massage is a specialty of Ayurveda. Marmas are important vital areas on the body, much like the acupuncture points of traditional Chinese medicine. The most important difference between acupuncture points and marmas is their size, with the marma areas being larger than acupuncture points. Marmas are also unlike acupuncture points in that they are not related to meridians. Additionally marma locations vary slightly from person to person.

By massaging marma areas, functions of the body and mind can be controlled and treated. Marma therapy is an important way in which to work on Prana, the life force in the body. Prana, as the main energy in the body, is directly related to the Vata dosha. Vata is the most important factor in the development and treatment of disease, and thus marma therapy is a direct method for disease prevention and treatment.

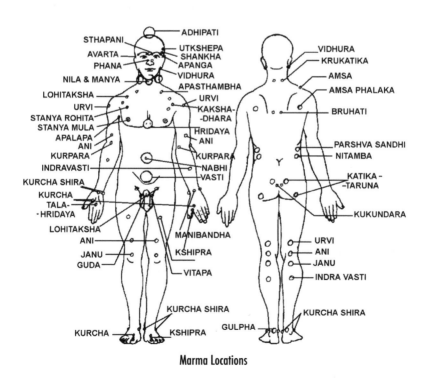

Marma Locations

Each marma relates to certain organs and systems. Marma therapy can be used to reduce aggravated doshas, reduce excess tissue growth, detoxification, or strengthening and tonification of tissues or organs.

There are many methods of treating marmas. These include massage with oils, application of herbal pastes (lepa chikitsa), application of plant alkalis (kshara karma), acupuncture (suchi karma), acupressure (mardana) application of heat (agni karma) - for stimulating and cleansing, or application of cold - for inflamation and bleeding, yoga postures (asanas) or yogic breathing techniques (pranayama).

The size of the marma areas are measured in anguli parimana, which are finger units relative to each individual. To determine anguli, the fingers of both hands, thumbs not included, are held side by side, the distance at the base of the fingers from one side to the other measured, and this distance is divided by eight. This measurement is one anguli.

Traditionally there are 107 defined marma areas on the body. Knowledge of these 107 sensitive anatomical areas was used in war for harming the enemy and also to protect oneself against injury. In therapy usually 21 main marma are used. The surgeon and author Sushruta elaborately discusses the marma areas. Knowledge of marma became an essential part of the training for surgeons, as injury to these points can produce death or disability. Modern day surgery mostly ignores these sensitive areas with resultant negative side effects. It has also been noted that vaccinations given in modern times can produce delayed, long term side effects if injected at certain marma areas on the body.

History of Marma

The origin of marma can be traced to the Saraswati culture which was located in the Indus valley of India. Knowledge of marma exists from the time of this ancient culture. The Saraswati culture produced the Vedas, which are some of the oldest known written records, dating back to 4000 BC. In the Vedas we find reference to items such as drapi, which is a type of body armor. In the Atharva-Veda we find reference to the term kavacha, which is a corselet or breastplate used for protection. In the great epic Mahabharata, we also find many references for marma (Karnaparva 19.31, Shalyaparva 32.63 and 36.64, Dronaparva 125.17, Bhishmaparva 95.47, Virataparva 31.12 and 15). It is interesting to note that there are also references to protective clothing for the marmas of elephants and horses. The Arthashastra of Kautilya, considered one of the best books for explaining money and politics, mentions the use of arrowheads made of metal along with an explanation of protective instruments which can be used to prevent injury to the marmas.

Modern day excavations at the ancient Indus valley cities of Harrappa and Mohenjodaro indicate that people in this culture were using various types of weapons in war. Axes, spears, daggers, maces and bows and arrows, made of copper or bronze, have been found in these excavations. To protect themselves from injury by these weapons they used knowledge of these vital marma areas.

Definition of Marma

Marma areas have been described by various texts and authors. According to the author Sushruta, marmas are defined as anatomical sites where muscles (mamsa), veins (sira), ligaments (snayu), bones (asthi) and joints (sandhi) meet together (Su.sh6/2). This does not mean that all these structures must be present at the site of the marma.

According to the Ashtanga Hridaya text, marmas are areas where important nerves (dhamani) come together along with other structures like muscles, tendons, etc. Vagbhata, the author, says that those sites which are painful, severely tender and show abnormal pulsation should also be considered as marma or vital points (A.H.sh. 4/37). These areas are the seats of "life" (A.H. sh. 4/ 2). They are the sites where not only the tridosha (Vata, Pitta and Kapha) are present, but also their subtle forms, i.e. Prana, Ojas (soma) and Tejas (agni), are also present with sattva, rajas and tamas - (Su. sh. 6 / 22, 45). Hence this is a specific area on the body, which has relation through Pranic channels to various internal organs.

According to another definition, marmas are "Marayanti iti Marmani'" (Dalhan) meaning these are the vital areas, some of which if injured, can produce death. If marmas are injured they do not always result in death, but can cause various diseases which are difficult to cure. (Uttara Rama Charita). Marmas can also be described as the junction of the body and the mind.

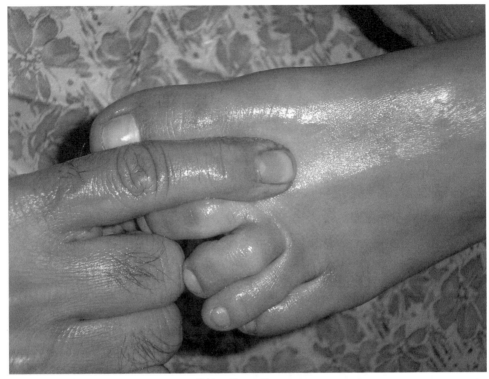

Kshipra Marma Massage

Various texts have described the number of marma in relation to anatomical structures differently as seen in the following tables.

According to the structure

	Asthanga Hridaya	Asthanga Sangraha	Sushruta Samhita
Mamsa	10	11	11
Sira	37	41	41
Snayu	23	27	27
Asthi	8	8	8
Sandhi	20	20	20
Dhamani	9	none	none
Total	107	107	107

According to the location

Legs (Sakthi)	22
Abdomen (Udara) and Chest (Ura)	12
Arms (Bahu)	22
Back (Prushtha)	14
Above the clavicle/collar bone (jatru-urdhva)	37
Total	107

According to size

One finger breadth (Anguli Parimana)	12
Two finger breadths	6
Three finger breadths	4
Fist size or Four finger breadths	29
One Half finger breadth	56
Total	107

According to the symptoms when injured

Sadyah Pranahara	19
Kalantara Pranahara	33
Vishalyaghna	3
Vaikalyakara	44
Rujakara	o8
Total	107

Marma Massage Technique

All the marmas are very sensitive areas and massage at these areas should be done gently. The massage should not be painful. The marmas on the head and abdomen are especially sensitive. Usually the thumb is used. The knuckle, wrist, palm and heel of the foot are also used in specific therapy. The massage should be done clockwise when tonification or strengthening of organs or tissues is required. To reduce aggravated doshas, reduce excess tissue growth, or detoxification, the massage should be done counter clockwise. Clockwise or counter clockwise can be determined by imagining a clock being placed on the body of the patient, then following the movement of the clock.

The marma massage should be performed for 5 minutes, twice a day. First apply steady pressure to the marma for 1 to 2 minutes. Follow with gentle massage to the area for another 3 to 4 minutes.

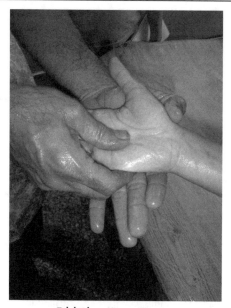

Talahridaya Marma Massage

Oils for Marma Massage

Various heavy or aromatic oils can be used for marma massage. Heavy oils include to oils such as sesame, coconut, olive, mustard, etc. Aromatic oils are also referred to as essential oils. The oils can either be removed after the marma massage or left remaining. The heavy oils are applied to the marma and massage is given as above. The essential oils can be used either with or without giving massage after they are applied. The application of essential oils to marmas without massage is a quick treatment when time is limited. Medicated heavy oils can also be used for marma massage. Medicated oils can be prepared one of two ways. One method is by mixing 1 ounce of heavy oil with 5 to 10 drops of essential oil. Another method is to make a strong decoction by boiling an herb in water, then adding this decoction to a heavy oil and boiling the mixture until the water has evaporated.

Three Important Marma Areas

Charaka has written a special chapter, trimarmiya adhyaya, in which he has mentioned that there are three important marmas. These are adhipati, hridaya and basti marmas Adhipati is located on the head (shira) at the vortex or very top of the head. Hridaya is located on the front of the chest, slightly towards the left side, between the second and the sixth intercostal space at the area of the heart. The marma area of hridaya is the size of the fist of the individual. This is also the size of the individuals heart. Basti is close to the symphisis pubis bone on the abdomen, below the navel.

Although different marmas on the body are connected to various doshas and subdoshas, generally these three main marmas relate to the three doshas, Vata, Pitta and Kapha. Basti relates to Vata, Hridaya to Pitta and Adhipati to Kapha.

Specific oils are used for specific marmas. The following oils can be used for marma massage to the three important marmas as explained by Charaka.

MARMA	HEAVY OIL	ESSENTIAL OIL
Basti	Sesame, olive, almond	Basil, cedar, cinnamon, clove, geranium, jasmine, lavender, myrrh, musk, orange, sage
Hridaya	Coconut, sunflower, sandalwood	Chamomile, cinnamon, gardenia, honeysuckle, lotus, mint, rose, saffron
Adhipati	Mustard, sesame, corn, jojoba	Basil, camphor, clove, eucalyptus, juniper, frankincense, lemon, marjoram, musk, myrrh, peppermint, rosemary, sage

Those who are interested in further studies of marma including detailed anatomical locations and therapy should read the book "Ayurveda and Marma Therapy" by Dr. Subhash Ranade, Dr. Avinash Lele and Dr. David Frawley, published by Lotus Press.

CHAPTER 11

SPECIALIZED AYURVEDIC MASSAGE TECHNIQUES

Shiro Abhyanga or Head Massage

The head is the center of the whole nervous system. Many important structures like the cerebrum, cerebellum, mid brain, and the sense organs such as the eyes, nose, ears and tongue are located in the head. Massage of the head provides nourishment to all these vital organs and promotes their natural and normal functions.

There are three very important areas on the head. Head massage should be done very carefully to these three areas.

1) The first area is at the top of the cranium, the anterior fontanel. This is called brahmarandhra in yoga and is also known as the "tenth gate". The brahmarandhra is a soft area at birth and later on becomes hard. A pad with oil is put on this spot after birth.

2) The second area is at the cowlick. The hairs at this area are turning in the form of a whirl either clockwise or counter clockwise. This area is also known as the crest or shikha.

3) The third area is where the neck meets the skull, the place of the brain stem or medulla oblongata.
   While doing massage on the head, these three areas should be carefully massaged. No patting, pounding or kneading is done on the head. Head massage is particularly beneficial before bathing in the morning to gently awaken the nerves.

Head massage is especially useful for the following

Prevents and cures headaches.
Prevents and cures hair loss by making the hair roots very strong.
Prevents and cures premature graying of hair.
Prevents and cures baldness.
Makes the hair long, soft and glossy.
Prevents and cures refraction errors of the eyes.
Endows a person with sound sleep.
Auto, or self head massage done in the evening helps remove the stress of the day and promotes peaceful sleep.

Technique for Head Massage

Start by pouring oil on the top of the head. This oil is then spread all over the head down to the temples using the fingers. For hair loss and other problems of the hair, the strokes should go from the top of the head downwards. Try to go along the seemanta marma areas and massage the scalp. Next, additional oil is poured on the cowlick (shikha marma). Continue rubbing this oil all over the head, twisting the hair in a clockwise direction at the roots. Lastly, gently press the head between both hands, simultaneously moving one hand forward and the other backward, then repeating.

When oil is applied to the head it gets absorbed into the scalp and reaches to the roots of the hair. This nourishes, lubricates and strengthens the hair roots and skin of the scalp, preventing hair loss and premature graying. It helps to improve circulation to the head and relaxes the muscles and nerve fibers. This helps to refresh both the mind and the body, relieving tension and fatigue. Massage to the head improves circulation of spinal fluid around the brain and spinal cord. It also increases the release of hormones and enzymes necessary for the growth of the brain and relaxation of the body. Additionally, massage to the head increases Prana, the subtle aspect of Vata dosha in the body. Massage to the eyebrows and forehead improves eyesight and the power of concentration. Head massage should be included in our daily health schedule.

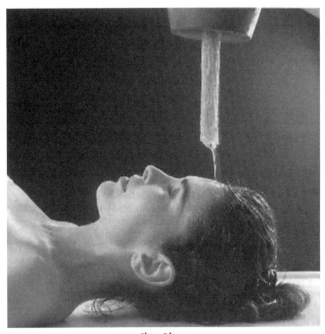

Shiro Dhara

Shiro Dhara

Shiro dhara is a process of running a fine stream of warm liquid on the head or forehead. It is one of the excellent therapies for diseases connected with the head, neck, eyes, ears, nose, throat and nervous system. Its therapeutic utility is proven for Vata alleviation and for patients suffering from Vata diseases such as insomnia and various mental disturbances. It is also used along with other medicines for patients suffering from epileptic fits. During this therapy, medicated oil, milk or buttermilk is poured on the forehead between the eyebrows.

If oil is used, this therapy is called taila dhara.

If milk is used, this therapy is called dugdha dhara.

If buttermilk is used, this therapy is called takra dhara.

Technique
Taila dhara

The patient lies on his back on a wooden table, called a droni, prepared specially for this therapy. First abhyanga is done to the head. The patient's head is made to rest in a slightly elevated position using a circular pillow. The physician selects the oil to be used. For holding the oil, a special vessel is prepared with a small hole in the bottom. The vessel is hung above the patient's head Oil is poured in the vessel and arranged so that the stream of oil is constant on the head. This therapy is given daily for 7 to 14 days and should be given early in the morning.

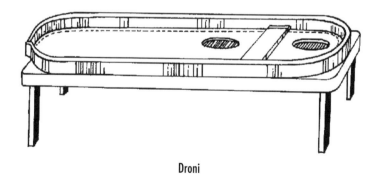

Droni

Dugdha Dhara

In this method a stream of milk is poured on the head. Medicated milk is used and is prepared by cooking the milk with bala (sida cordifolia) and shatavari (asperagus racemosus). This is very useful for patients suffering from insanity, sleeplessness, giddiness and burning sensations.

Takra Dhara

This therapy is useful for premature graying of the hair, fatigue, headache, giddiness and burning sensation to the palms and sole of the feet, as well as for different types of disease of ear, nose and eyes.

For this procedure a mixture of buttermilk with a decoction of amalaki is used. The buttermilk should be the type as specified in Ayurveda. Most buttermilk sold in stores is not the correct type for this procedure. To prepare the buttermilk as specified in Ayurveda, first bring milk to boiling. Remove the milk and allow it to cool. After it has cooled add yogurt culture, or a few drops of lemon juice if yogurt culture is not available. Keep the mixture in a warm place overnight. The next day the yogurt will be done. Put the yogurt mixture into a blender and churn for two minutes. The mix will separate into butter and a remaining clearer mixture of buttermilk. The buttermilk is very light and will invigorate agni, the digestive fire.

All types of dhara, whether they use oil, milk or buttermilk, are beneficial as follows -
1. Alleviation of doshas in the region of the head, neck, eyes, ear and nose.
2. Improving the functions of the brain and the central nervous system.
3. Maintaining calm and quietness of the mind.
4. Reducing stress and strain.

Shiro Basti

Shiro basti involves keeping oil over the head with the help of a tubular leather cap that is filled with oil. This is one of the more important external oleation methods. It is indicated in facial palsy, insomnia, dry nose, dry eyes, dry mouth, migraine headache, loss of memory, mental stress and strain and in Vata vitiation (increase) as well as Vata diseases.

Preliminary procedure

It is preferable to first shave the scalp. The procedure may be performed without shaving. Give a gentle massage to the scalp and forehead, then mild fomentation to the scalp, head and neck.

Main Procedure

Place the leather cap over the head down to the top of ears. Fill the gap between the head and cap with wheat dough. Plastic mud can also been used for this purpose. Put warm sesame oil gradually in the cap. It should be filled to at least 4 inches above the scalp. This oil should be retained in the cap for 50 minutes in Vata vitiation, 40 minutes in Pitta vitiation and 30 minutes in Kapha vitiation, or until signs of optimum treatment are noted.

Optimum signs of the procedure are secretions from the nose and mouth along with alleviation of the symptoms for which the procedure is undertaken. Once these signs are noted, the oil is removed from cap and the cap is then removed.

Post procedure

After removal of the cap, ask the patient to take a warm water bath. Advise the patient to avoid exposure to excessive cold, heat or dampness and to keep the head covered with a hat if they are outside in cold weather. Usually this procedure is done for 7 consecutive days.

Netra tarpana/Netra basti

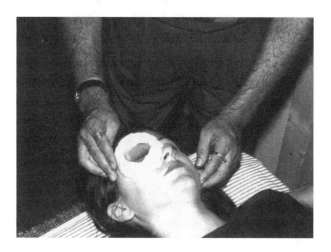

Netra tarpana, or netri basti, means bathing the eye with medicated oil. It is an ancient treatment from Ayurveda to release tension and to treat various eye diseases This treatment is used to improve visual power as well as for the treatment of various other diseases like ptosis (drooping of the upper eyelid), paresis (partial paralysis) of the muscles of the eye, squint due to muscular palsy, etc. We have found that it also brings luster to the eyes, relieves dryness of the conjunctiva, excessive blinking of the eye lids, enhances color and visual perception and creates a sense of ease in the region of the eye. Due to constant work with computers along with excessive exposure to bright light and television, there is stress and strain on the eyes which become fatigued and tired very easily. For such problems Netra tarpana is an extremely beneficial treatment. This treatment should be done in a calm, quiet and protected environment.

Requirements

Table, vessel containing medicated oil, vessel containing black gram flour or wheat flour.

Preliminary procedure

First give a gentle massage to the face, eyebrows and eyes using very little oil.

Main procedure

Form a round ring about 1 1/2 inches in height, around the eye socket using black gram or wheat dough. Pour warm cows ghee or medicated (triphala) cows ghee into the ring. Ask the patient to regularly open and close the eye four or five times per minute.

For Vata vitiation bathe the eye in the ghee for 60 minutes. For Pitta vitiation 40 minutes, for Kapha 20 minutes. Afterwards remove the ghee by making a small indentation on outer edge of the dough ring and allow the ghee to drain. If required carry out the process for both eyes at the same time.

Post procedure

After the treatment, wipe around the eye with a soft cloth and ask the patient to keep away from bright light for half an hour. This procedure can be repeated for 7 days.

Ear Massage

Points on the outer ear are considered to represent organs in the body and massaging these point on the ear affects the corresponding body organs. External massage to the outer area of the ear is also useful for treating various ear diseases.

Karna Purana

Karna Purana is a technique where the ears are filled with oil. The ears are a main location of Vata, and putting sesame oil in the ear treats Vata in the region above the clavicle. By pouring oil into the ears we can improve the function of the ear and also treat diseases specific to the ears such as earache, deafness and tinnitus (a buzzing or ringing in the ears). Diseases of nearby organs such as headache, lock-jaw or giddiness, receding gums, painful conditions of the teeth and wax in the ear can also be treated.

In the case of wax in the ear or hearing loss use sesame oil. For earache use garlic oil (garlic cooked in sesame oil) and for tinnitus use coconut oil. For receding gums use bala (sida cordifolia) cooked in sesame oil.

The ears and eyes are both closely related to the soles of the feet. Pouring oil into the ears produces coolness and removes burning sensations in the feet. Pouring of oil in the ear should be done before meals during the daytime.

Technique

Hold the earlobe between the thumb and index finger. Give a rolling and gentle squeezing massage, using oil, to the outer edge of the ear. Also apply oil to the lobe. Next, pour warm oil, according to the condition being treated, into the ear and rub the ear for a few seconds. Repeat the procedure in other ear. Do not put oil into the ears more than two times per week.

Benefits

Facilitates improvement in circulation of the ear.
Helps to balance Vata dosha by having an indirect effect on colon.
Stimulates the brain.
Lowers blood pressure.
Absence of stiffness in chin and neck.
Absence of all ear diseases.
Removes dust and germs from the inner ear.

CAUTION - If there is an ear infection, perforation of the eardrum or a pus discharge from the ear (the ear should be dry inside) do not put oil into the ear. If you are unsure, or if there is a history of a ruptured ear drum, do not put anything into the ear. Garlic oil in the ear may be permissible to treat an ear infection, but only if the eardrum is intact.

Nasya

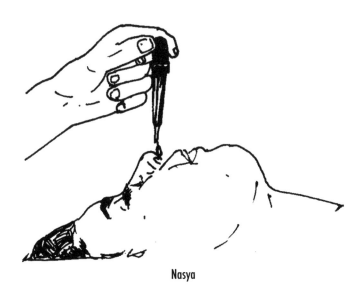

Nasya

Nasya means nasal administration of medicated powders or liquids. It is a procedure in which medication is administered through the nostrils in order to purify the head and neck region. Nasya should be given as a supportive treatment along with massage in this region. "Nasa hi shiraso dwaram" means the nose is a doorway to the head. Vitiated (abnormal) doshas above the region of the clavicle, in the head and neck area, are eliminated through the nose with this treatment. This therapy is specifically advised for the head and neck. Many diseases of the eyes, ears, neck, head and throat can be treated with Nasya. From the cosmetic point of view, Nasya reduces dark rings under the eyes and a sunken or puffy look around the eyes.

Indications for Nasal medication

Headache, migraine, stiffness in the head, neck or shoulders, lock-jaw, dental pain, nasal pain, eye pain, sinusitis, facial paralysis, epilepsy, sleeplessness or loss of speech. In short, any diseases of the nose, eye, ear and throat. Medicines used for this purpose are oils, pastes, powders, plant juices, decoctions, infusions and smoking of herbs.

Contra indications for Nasya

Pregnancy, menstruation, after a hot bath, after eating, after sexual interaction or after drinking alcohol.

Types of Nasya
Cleansing Nasya (Shodhana nasya)

In this type of nasya, hot and penetrating powders or oils are used. Due to their irritating nature they eliminate doshas from the region

Pacifying nasya (Shamana nasya)

In this type of nasya medicated ghee or oil is used. This reduces the doshas but does not eliminate them completely.

Tonification nasya (Brimhana nasya)

This is used for nourishing the tissues. Ghee or oil which is medicated with herbs such as shatavari or ashwaghanda is used.

Technique
Pre procedure

Apply a suitable oil on the face, forehead, shoulder and nasal region and give wet or dry fomentation (heating) to this region. Allow the patient to lie on their back and ask them to tilt their head back so that the nose is pointed upwards towards the ceiling.

Main procedure

Put 4 to 8 drops of warm oil, juice or decoction in the right nostril. Close the opposite nostril and ask the patient to inhale the oil or medicine. Repeat with the left nostril.

Post procedure

Ask the patient to remain with their nose pointed upwards towards the ceiling for 10 seconds, then have them rest on their back with the head in a normal position. If the oil or medicine moves into the throat they can either swallow or spit it out.

Pradhamana Nasya

Pradhamana is a specific type of nasya which is used mainly for purification purpose. A special apparatus is available for this purpose which has a main container with a nozzle and a rubber bulb attached. Powder or liquid medicine is put into the main container. The nozzle is put into the nostril after following steps a and b above. The rubber bulb is squeezed to administer approximately 125 mg of medication into the nostril. The medicines used for this purpose are usually of a hot potency and of a penetrating quality and nasal secretions will start immediately. After the signs of proper purification, such as lightness in the head and body, let the patient rest.

Vapor Nasya

In vapor nasya a decoction of herbs is brought to a boil. The decoction is allowed to remain boiling and the patient leans over the boiling medicine, covering their head with a towel, and inhales the vapor.

Benefits

Elimination of vitiated (abnormal) doshas through the nose. Lightness in the head and body, good sleep, proper functioning of the sense organs and the mind, and relief of symptoms for which nasya is indicated.

Foot Massage (Padabhyanga)

Padabhyanga means foot massage. Padabhyanga is highly praised in Ayurveda. Before going to bed it is very beneficial to massage the soles of the feet. It is relaxing and promotes sound sleep. Foot massage every day protects us from diseases of the eyes along with other vital organs such as the heart, kidneys and brain and is considered to bring peace, prosperity and good luck. According to ancient Ayurvedic scriptures, "diseases do not go near one who massages his feet before sleeping just as snakes do not approach eagles". One should carry out foot massage for treating dryness, numbness, roughness, fatigue, lack of sensation and cracking in the feet. Foot massage promotes strength for walking and running, and gives sturdiness to the limbs.

A beneficial description of the effects of foot massage is written by Vagbhata. According to Vagbhata there are four important nerves in the sole of the foot which are connected to the head. Due to heat, friction and excessive pressure on the feet, these nerves are affected with a result of reduced eyesight. It is said that a person who receives regular massage to the soles of the feet never suffers from eye diseases. An important basic principle is that the feet (karmendriya) and the eyes (dnyanendriya) are both related to the element of fire. Although the feet and the eyes are located far apart from each other they are interconnected.

It is advisable to apply castor oil to the sole of the foot and then massage the foot with the bottom of a copper vessel. Castor oil, although heating, is specified in the classical Ayurvedic texts for use in foot massage with a copper vessel. A copper vessel is used because the copper will absorb heat from the body. If castor oil is not available, coconut oil can be used. This is extremely beneficial in the case of burning eyes due to excessive walking in the sun. This is also beneficial for those who work around heat sources or masseurs who absorb negative energy from their clients.

A simple mustard oil massage will prevent cold weather cracking and peeling of the skin on the feet. Mustard oil also reduces and eliminates infections caused by fungus and bacteria. When a foot massage is not possible, simply bathing the feet with cool water produces freshness in the whole body.

Benefits of foot massage

Foot massage provides increased foot strength and the ability to stand continuously for long periods. With foot massage one can avoid hardness, stiffness, roughness and tiredness in the entire body. It is also beneficial for treating cracks in the soles of the feet, varicose veins and for improvement in eyesight. The kurcha marma, located on the sole of the foot, is very important for treatment of the eyes. Proper foot massage also helps produce a sound sleep.

The science of Reflexology states that the sole of the foot has connections with various organs of the body. Proper foot massage at the respective site on the foot, with specific oils, prevents and cures various diseases. According to the science of Reflexology, various organs such as the heart, lungs, kidney, brain and intestines all can be stimulated by foot massage.

Vertebral Column Massage

The vertebral column is one of the main seats of tarpaka and avalambaka Kapha. Tarpaka Kapha is located nearer to the spinal chord while Avalambaka Kapha is located around the muscles surrounding the vertebra. The vertebral column is closely related to asthi (bones) and majja (bone marrow and nerve tissue), Prana and Vyana Vata and Sadhaka Pitta.

There are 33 vertebrae, of which 24 are moveable. The moveable vertebrae consists of 7 cervical, 12 thoracic and 5 lumbar. The remaining 9 vertebrae are located in the sacrum and the coccyx, and are fixed. Between each vertebrae there is a disc, and nerves pass through openings in the vertebrae.

Every masseur must know the anatomy and physiology of the spine. If the spine is properly aligned and strong, the vital life force will flow properly and all body functions will work smoothly. Massage of the spine can cure many bodily and some psychic disorders. Regular massage to the spine can slowly bring about a change in the body and the mind.

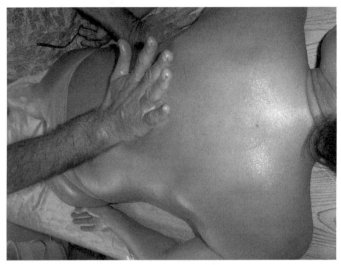

Spinal Chord Massage

Massage to the spine must include oil and pressure. The proper oil and the proper pressure on the vertebrae and surrounding muscles is required. To begin the massage, oil is applied to the whole back. Start from the cervical region placing the thumbs on both sides of each vertebra. Massage each vertebra and the surrounding muscles, slowly moving down the spine. While massaging the vertebrae feel for areas which are tender or painful. The entire spinal column massage should last for about 15 minutes.

Benefits
Relief of stiffness and back pain.
Proper functioning of the nervous system.
Release of tension in the mind.

Spinal Column Exercise
Twisting of the spine to the right and left is the best exercise for the spinal column. The twisting increases the circulation of the spinal fluid. Twisting of the spine can be done by laying on the back and lifting both legs to a straight up position. Slowly lower both legs to the right, touching the floor momentarily Then bring the legs back to a straight up position and lower both legs to the left, again touching the floor momentarily. Repeat this series of touching to the right, then left, 5 times.

Kundalini Massage
The human spine is a seat of miracles. The central nervous system and the autonomous nervous system both work through the spine. The spine is a seat of all the chakras (psychic centers) except the sixth chakra. Yoga and

Tantra, the sciences that deal with the evolution of human consciousness, are full of descriptions of the mysterious powers of Kundalini. Kundalini, the serpent power that operates through the spine, lies at the base of the vertebral column, in the root chakra. Kundalini is the seed energy of the subtle body. Kundalini contains within itself all the power of consciousness. Kundalini massage is a very ancient art of massage. This type of massage is practiced in many yoga schools in India.

Dr. David Frawley in his book "From the River of Heaven", has explained that Kundalini can be recognized as an intense power of devotion or attention. This is related with Yoga of devotion and Yoga of knowledge. The proper awakening of Kundalini is through divine grace. This does not mean that effort on our part is not useful, but that our effort must be to attune ourselves to this grace. If artificial methods, like Kundalini massage or willful, forced or egoistic practices are used, there can be possible side effects. It is advisable that Kundalini massage be done under supervision and with proper care. The premature arousing of Kundalini can burn up the nervous system and can limit or prevent our spiritual growth permanently. The arousing of the Kundalini is usually brought about through coordination of posture, massage, breath and mantra.

For Kundalini massage the proper medicated oil should be used. The patient is asked to lie on their abdomen. The massage is started at the bottom of the spine, moving upwards. An alternate method of Kundalini massage uses different oils at different chakras instead of only one oil for the entire massage.

Lymph Drainage Massage

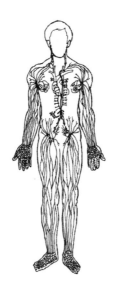

Lymphatic System

Lymph drainage massage works directly with the three circulatory systems of the body simultaneously. The three circulatory systems which are involved are the blood vascular system, the lymphatic system and the nervous system. The lymphatic system is the one which is most directly involved in the massage. The lymphatic system works through ducts, nodes and passages. This lymphatic system is a supplementary system to the blood vascular system. It runs side by side with the blood vascular system and through osmosis gets mixed with the blood and supplied to the whole body. The lymphatic system assists the blood circulation by draining excess fluids from the blood stream, easing the workload of the heart. It also offers an alternative route for the return of tissue fluids to the blood stream.

The masseur must remember that the lymph nodes which produce lymphatic fluid are located underneath all the joints of the body. By rubbing and applying circular movements to the joints, one can stimulated these lymph nodes. Pressure, fomentation and deep breathing exercises can also stimulate the lymph system. Increasing lymph flow reduces blood pressure. This is one of the reasons massage is given to patients with high blood pressure. The lymphatic massage may be particularly useful when employed in a preventive health care system. Lymphatic massage causes a number of subjective changes in mood. It is a painless massage and is also associated with the marmas (vital areas). Lymph massage can be done with simple heavy oil, with a mixture of heavy and aromatic oils, or with any Ayurvedic medicated oil.

Massage for Relaxation

For relaxation, massage should be done very gently. In cases of mental or physical strain, anxiety, worries, insomnia, weakness of muscles, cramps and old age, massage should also be performed very gently. Massage of the spine, shoulder, leg and hands helps in these cases.

CHAPTER 12

MASSAGE FOR BEAUTY

Beauty massage consists of the following types of treatments.
1) Face massage.
2) Head and hair massage.
3) Eye massage.
4) Nail massage /nail care.

Face Massage

The following steps are used in Ayurvedic facial massage.
1) Cleansing.
2) Massage with oil.
3) Herbal steam or compress.
4) Gentle scrub.
5) Cleansing and nutrifying masks/facial packs.
6) Toning/rejuvenating.
7) Moisturizing.
8) Hydrating/mists.
9) (optional) Application of makeup.

Cleansing, toning and moisturizing should be done every day. It is advisable to carry out a full program once a week or at least twice a month.

Facial massage provides the following benefits.

Enhances the nourishment and cleansing of facial tissues which gives a glowing complexion to the face.

Maintains good tone and elasticity to all skin layers which helps to hold youthful contours.

Relieves facial tensions and bodily stress and helps to remove wrinkles.

Cleansing

Sweat and the accompanying waste products constantly come out on the surface of the skin attracting dirt and offering a home to bacteria. Initial cleansing removes this dirt, making the skin surface fresh and ready to receive a facial massage. Ayurveda suggests the use of herbal powders called ubtans to cleanse the skin. The powders are mixed with liquids and applied as a thin scrub. All of these herbal powders improve circulation, sooth the skin and bring a glow to the complexion. For this purpose, powders of coriander, manjishtha, nutmeg, tulsi or sandalwood are generally used. They can be mixed with spring water, milk or aloe juice. These powders can be mixed with aromatic oils of rose or sandalwood and then applied on the face. When mixed with oils these are referred to as an oil based cleanser

Massage with oil

Step one - Apply warm oil on both palms and start massaging with smooth strokes starting from the midline of the chin.

Step two - Place the fingers under the jaw, keeping the thumb on the jaw line. Ask the patient to open his mouth slightly and then manipulate the chin and jaw area by pressing up and releasing gently.

Step three - Place the thumbs on the jaw at the chin with the index and third finger underneath the jaw line. Apply pressure to the top and inner part of jawbone. Make light and small strokes in clockwise circles at the temples.

Step four - Place the index finger between lower lip and tip of the chin. Ask the patient to open his mouth and make small clockwise circles at these points. Continue the massage from the cheeks to the temples.

Step five - Place the tip of the index finger between nose and upper lip. This is the area of the shrungataka marma. Press gently. Then stroke from this point out, on both sides, down to the corners of the mouth. Then stroke under the cheek bones to the top of the ear, over the ear, at the base of the ear where it touches the head to the bony bump (mastoid) behind the earlobe. Pay attention to the vidhura marma located here.

Step six - Hold the side of the patient's head with the left hand. Place the right index finger just above the base of the nostril. Give a circular massage from this point moving slowly up to the bony prominence behind the ear lobe, going over the ear.

Step seven - Start massaging from a point midway between the outer corner of the eye and the tip of the nostrils. Give a circular massage from this point to the mastoid bone behind the ear going over the ear.

Step eight - Starting at the inner end of the eyebrow, pinch along the eyebrow to the outer edge using the index finger and thumb.

Step nine - Stroke from the tip of the nose to the area of the third eye, which is located between the eyebrows. This is the Sthapani marma. Massage this area with a gentle circular motion.

Step ten - Massage the forehead using zigzag motions from one side of the forehead to the other. Repeat this from right to left and left to right.

Different types of massage techniques such as pinching or pressure are given to all areas of the face. Using gentle vibrations to the face area also will give a soothing effect.

Very gentle friction is important in the case of giving massage to the eyebrows, ears and nose. For friction, sometimes a cotton or raw silk cloth is used

Herbal steam or compress

The warmth, moisture and fragrance of herbal steam melts away muscular tension. It also helps to calm the mind along with removing stress and strain. Using steam is one of the oldest traditions in Ayurveda. The moisture of the steam softens dry skin. The heat boosts facial circulation and activates the pores and glands, which brings dirt and toxins to the surface. To balance Vata dosha, oil can be applied after the steam. Frequency of steaming is determined by the condition of the skin

For dry skin, steaming should be done twice a week. It is advisable to mix dashamula, rose or sandalwood powder with water. For normal and oily skin, steaming should be done once a week. For normal skin, it is preferable to mix ashwagandha and sandalwood powder, while for oily skin, lemongrass and rose powder is beneficial.

For compresses prepare a decoction of herbs. Let the decoction cool slightly, and while the decoction is still warm dip a towel into the decoction and keep this compress on the body part being treated. This will put direct moist heat on the area and is useful for relief of pain and other symptoms.

Gentle scrubs

A scrub should be done very gently using a cotton cloth. It stimulates circulation and brings a glowing luster to the skin. A scrub is cleansing as it removes dead skin cells along with stimulating new skin growth.

Cleansing and nutrifying masks/facial packs

This extracts dirt from the deeper layers of the skin, preventing blackheads and acne. Muscles under the skin are nourished as they receive vitamins and minerals. Masks can also stimulate the deepest layer of the skin to make new growth. Clay is the best base for a mask (gopichandan or multani mitti is used). Clay is a rich source of minerals. Aloe vera juice, lemon juice, or spring water is mixed with the clay to prepare the mask.

Face packs are a thin paste, while face masks are thicker. They improve circulation as well as clean and tighten the facial skin. Fruits and vegetables like orange, cucumber and fresh fruit juices are used to make face packs. Both masks and face packs should be removed with cool water and a clean wash cloth.

Toning/rejuvenating

Toners are useful to remove the residue of all previous procedures and also tone the skin. Typically rose water or holy basil (tulsi) water is used as a toner.

For rejuvenating the skin a mixture of milk, saffron and honey can be applied. Almond oil with milk can also be used.

Moisturizing

All types of skin need moisturizing. Moisturizing protects the skin from heat and dry wind by acting as a physical barrier. It also protects the skin from invasion by bacteria. Aloe vera, with glycerin, butter, ghee etc. can be used as a moisturizer It is should preferably be applied at night.

Hydrating/mists

A gentle touch of a spray mist brings vitality back to the complexion any time of day. Mists are wonderful in a dry climate. Apply the mist before and after moisturizing to assist absorption. Mists are made up of pure spring water and sometimes contain gold or silver. To make gold or silver water for a mist, a heavy gold or silver ring can be boiled for 5 minutes in water. After cooling, the water can be used as a mist. Usually gold is used for Vata or Kapha constitutions, while silver is used for Pitta.

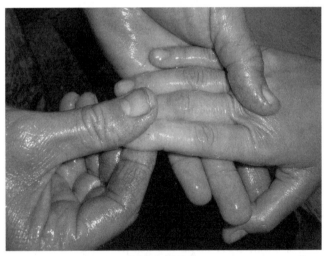

Massage for Nails

Nail Massage

Our nails are a byproduct (mala) of our bones (asthi dhatu). The state of our bones therefore may be reflected in our nails. Our nails can also be an indicator of the state of our body in general. Ridges, discolorations, dryness or cracking of the nails can be used as an indicator of the state of our tissues and doshas. The nails should be examined and weighed relative to the other bodily indicators as part of an overall patient diagnosis.

Vata type people have nails which tend to be irregular in shape with ridges running either the length of the nail or across the nail. These ridges are blackish in color. Pitta type nails are an even oval shape, soft, pink and smooth. Kapha nails are square, thick, hard and strong.

Healthy nails are pinkish in color, smooth and evenly shaped with a slight convexity White spots on the nails indicate calcium and zinc deficiency. Bitten nails indicate nervousness. Brittle nails indicate low iron or vitamin A. Yellowish nails may indicate jaundice. Bluish nails may indicate a lung and heart imbalance. Pale nails can indicate anemia. For healthy nails the diet should be rich in proteins, minerals such as iron and calcium, as well as vitamins D and A.

Regular massage to the nail beds is very important for the health of the nails. On a daily basis, dip the fingers in warm water, then using a very soft brush, clean the nails and fingers. Follow with a drop of sesame oil on the nail and nail base and massage very gently.

Application of herbal pastes, containing triphala, aloe gel and neem oil once a week to the nails and nail base is helpful in giving strength to the nails. Allow the paste to remain on for 20 minutes and then wash the nails with warm water and lemon juice in a proportion of 1 part water to 1/6 part lemon juice. This is helpful for nourishment of the nails and will give a shining appearance.

CHAPTER 13

MASSAGE FOR SPECIFIC DISEASES

Arthritis

Arthritis can be acute or chronic. In Ayurveda it is commonly known as Sandhivata. Sandhi means joint, and vitiation (increase) of Vata is usually the prominent factor in this disease. Acute arthritis can be a due to trauma, infections, gout or hemophilia. It can also be due to toxins, called ama. When this toxin mixes with a vitiated (abnormal) dosha, it can cause rheumatic arthritis (amavata). Chronic arthritis is usually a result of disorders of the immune system and vitiation of the doshas. Chronic arthritis can also be due to different infections, such as tuberculosis, as well as degenerative disorders.

Osteoarthritis

Osteoarthritis is called Asthigata Vata. This is a disease that usually occurs in people over 50 years of age. Affected joints are painful, and the patient also suffers from other symptoms of Vata vitiation such as insomnia, weakness and loss of strength in the muscles. Pitta and Kapha types also exist.

Treatment

Vata type - Massaging the joints with narayan oil, bala oil, or dhanvantari oil is very effective. When these oils are not available use simple sesame oil, or cook anti-arthritic herbs such as ashwagandha or galangal with sesame oil for external massage.

Pitta type - Massage with nimbamrutadi oil along with cold ice packs to the joint is useful.

Kapha type - Massage with vishagarbha oil helps to loosen the joints, detoxify the ama and improve the affected joint function. Prasarini oil is also useful.

Diet

Proper nutritive food with Vitamins A and D should be given. Natural calcium, which is available in many dairy products including cheese, milk, butter and ghee should be included. Natural calcium in the form of eggshell ash or coral calcium can also be used, $\frac{1}{4}$ tsp. of either, taken twice a day with ghee. Eggshell ash can be prepared by drying, crushing and heating eggshells in an iron pan until they are reduced to an ash. A preparation of five natural calciums, known as praval panchamrita, is also good. The dosage is 125 mg, twice a day, for one month. Plenty of leafy green vegetables should be included in the diet.

Rheumatic Arthritis

In Ayurveda rheumatic arthritis is called amavata. A low digestive fire produces toxins (ama) in the digestive tract, which then circulate through the entire body via the heart and blood vessels causing fever, heart disorders, joint problems and other serious complications. Therefore, when ama is present in the digestive system, one should never carry out excessive exercise which would circulate these toxins throughout the body. Signs of ama in the digestive system are a coating on the tongue which does not scrape off and a stool which does not float in water. It is said that rheumatic arthritis "bites the joints and leaks the heart". The disease starts in the stomach and spreads to the joints and heart. The joints are one of the main sites of Kapha dosha. Shleshaka Kapha, a subtype of Kapha, is the synovial fluid in the joints. Ama and Kapha have similar properties and therefore ama tends to gravitate to the Kapha dosha sites in the body such as the joints.

Symptoms

The main symptom of this disease is a fleeting type of pain in the big joints. The inflammation and pain shifts from joint to joint very rapidly. In the acute stage, the big joints are inflamed on a given day and then absolutely normal the next day when some other joint becomes affected. When the heart gets involved usually the mitral valve is affected and there is either stenosis or a regurgitation type deformity.

Ama stage

In this stage the joints are inflamed, swollen and very painful. Application of prasarani oil helps to relieve severe pain in this acute condition. Until the ama is detoxified, the patient should take only warm vegetable soup. Whenever the patient is thirsty they should drink warm water or herbal tea. When ama is present massage to the inflamed joints is contraindicated.

Treatment

To destroy ama, fasting should be carried out in the acute stage. The swollen joints should be fomented using dry heat which liquefies the ama in the joint. Hot sand in a bolus is best. Electrical pads or infared lamps may also be used. One teaspoon of castor oil should be taken internally with ginger tea, which will detoxify the ama in 3 to 4 days.

Nirama stage

Nirama means without ama. When the ama gets detoxified, this "no ama" stage is present. In this stage the swelling of the joints disappears but they are still very painful.

Massage

Use sahacharadi oil, rasona oil or saindhavadi oil for massage. During this stage the patient can take a light diet which will not put out the digestive fire. Broth of white meat (chicken or turkey), basmati rice, ghee, buttermilk or milk and plenty of fruit juice can be taken along with green vegetables.

Rheumatoid Arthritis

Vitiated (abnormal) Vata affects the joints and produces this disease. This is also known as 'Sandhigata Vata'. The small and large joints are affected and become painful and swollen. If it is not treated properly it becomes chronic and deformity may develop in the affected joints. People over 40 are affected most often. It is a systemic connective tissue disorder affecting the joints and muscle wasting and inflammation of the muscles around the joints is very common.

Symptoms

In a typical Vata type of rheumatoid arthritis the pain is throbbing, migrating and cutting. It is relieved by fomentation. Deformity is more likely to take place. Other symptoms of Vata aggravation like constipation, gas, nervousness and insomnia are common. Pitta and Kapha types also exist. Pitta types are more inflamed, red, hot to the touch and are accompanied with fever, thirst and irritability. In Pitta types, pain increases by fomentation. In the Kapha type there is more swelling and edema around the joints, and the pain is a dull aching type which is relieved by fomentation.

Treatment

Vata type - Affected joints should be massaged with sahacharadi oil and then given fomentation with medicated vapor of herbs like holy basil (tulsi -ocimum sanctum).

Pitta type - Massage with kottamchukadi oil. A preparation called chandanbalalakshadi oil is also useful in this condition.

Kapha type - For massage, a light application of dhanvantara oil is indicated. If there is a lot of pain and swelling, dry fomentation by infrared lamp or heated sandbag is beneficial.

Traumatic Arthritis

Vata vitiation is the predominant factor in the pathogenesis. If there are no visible injuries on the skin, an external application of curcuma amada with lime is beneficial

Massage

Apply Vishgarbha oil and then carry out fomentation of the affected joint.

Backache

Although pain anywhere in the back is known as backache, usually it is connected to the vertebral column or the attached muscles. Backache is very common after 40 both in males and females.

Causative Factors

Various diseases of the vertebral column, spinal cord and meninges diseases, fibrosis, lumbago, slipped disks and other diseases of the abdominal and pelvic organs are causative factors. Lack of calcium after delivery, obesity, tubercular infections, fractures and tumors can also be responsible. In modern times defective posture, stress and lifting of heavy articles are primary causes.

Treatment

Vata vitiation, bone and muscle weakness are the major factors to consider when providing treatment.

Massage

Mahamasha oil followed by mild fomentation or a warm bath.

Technique

Before starting the treatment, make sure that the patient does not suffer from a "slipped disc". The back muscles are very strong and the masseur will have to work deep and with a lot of pressure on these muscles as well as the vertebrae. The pressure can further damage a slipped disk.

It is advisable to start the treatment with effleurage over the lumbar muscles. Follow with light strokes so that the muscles will relax properly. Next use petrissage and a firm kneading type of massage. Lastly, tapotment strokes should be given.

Since this is a Vata disorder, Panchakarma procedures such as alternate cleansing enemas and oil enemas are beneficial. For the oil enema, 60 to 70 ml. of sesame oil should be used and it should be given preferably in the evening. Courses of alternating oil enemas (anuvasana basti) and medicated cleansing enemas (niruha basti) continuing for 7, 10, or 15 days should be given.

Cervical Spondylitis

Spondyl denotes vertebrae or the spine. When there is inflammation of the ligaments and muscles surrounding the vertebrae this disorder is produced. This is a high Vata and Pitta disorder.

Causative factors

As our age increases, there is a natural tendency of wear and tear of the vertebrae. When they become weakened through this wear they can become easily afflicted by inflammation. Causes like trauma due to constant shocks by heavy equipment or bad road surfaces, or incorrect posture such as bending the neck while typing, writing or reading is also responsible for this problem.

Symptoms

Most commonly the cervical vertebrae are affected. There is pain in the neck that may radiate towards the hands and fingers. Pain may be at the back near the scapular region. Tingling and numbness in the hands is very common. Vertigo after bending the neck may be present.

Treatment

It is useful to try the following mixture for three weeks: 2 teaspoons Castor oil, 2 teaspoons fresh ginger juice, 1/4 teaspoon lemon juice and 1 teaspoon ghee taken on an empty stomach early in the morning. This is an ancient anti Vata formula that is Vyadhi Pratyanik, meaning disease specific. It is also very important to observe the correct postures while writing, typing, etc. Forward bending of the neck should be avoided. While sleeping care should be taken that the pillow is not too thick. A larger pillow causes the neck to remain more in a forward bending position which increases the problem.

Massage

The best oil is prabhanjana vimardana. If this is not available use dhanvantara oil or plain sesame oil. It should be followed by nadi sweda fomentation with a mixture of water and a few drops of eucalyptus oil or leaves of vitex negundo . Nadi sweda is a technique where a small rubber tube is attached to a pressure cooker and the steam directed at the area being heated.

Technique

The neck contains many vital arteries and veins which are connected to the brain. Caution must be taken while massaging the front portion of the neck. Undue pressure on the carotid arteries can cause serious trouble in the heart and other circulatory disturbances.

The back portion of the neck has cervical vertebrae and various muscles and ligaments attached to it. The masseur should massage these muscles in a downward direction (the pressure should be on the down stroke).

Constipation

Bowel movements differ from individual to individual. They depend on the type of diet and the general activity of the person. However, constipation can be defined as an accumulation of toxins (ama) in the colon due to a lack of bowel movement. Ideally, one should have an easy bowel movement in the early morning and the stool should float on the water. If the stool sinks, is sticky, or has a very bad smell it indicates the presence of toxins (ama) in the colon. The coating on the tongue also indicates if there is ama in the system as the tongue is a mirror of our digestion. Usually the tongue has a thin, slightly whitish coating when we first wake up in the morning. After scraping the tongue (a practice that should be done in addition to brushing the teeth every morning) this coating should disappear. If the coating remains, this indicates toxins in the digestive tract. The heavier the coating the more toxins (ama) is in the system. Ama is one of the main factors in the disease process.

Symptoms of constipation may include gas, pain in the abdomen, bloating, headache, insomnia and uneasiness.

Causative factors

Developing the proper urge in the morning is very important. The modern lifestyle of getting up late and rushing to work does not allow this habit to develop, which can lead to constipation. Many people with a Vata constitution suffer from constipation. The main cause is dietary. Eating a meal after sundown or eating food that is hard to digest produces toxins (ama) in the colon. Food without roughage, too much coffee and tea, eating legumes (dried peas or beans), dry foods, very cold drinks and smoking all contribute to constipation.

Acute constipation

For immediate relief, give an enema using 60 to 70 ml. of warm sesame oil. Massage the abdomen with sesame oil and carry out light fomentation of the abdomen. If this is not possible use a glycerin suppository. If the tongue has a heavy coating it means that there are a lot of toxins in the colon. Fasting, anti ama diets and herbs to detoxify the ama should be given. When the digestion has improved give strong purgatives like senna, rhubarb or castor oil.

Chronic constipation

Habit forming allopathic laxatives or purgatives cannot treat chronic constipation because constant use of purgatives creates dryness in the colon that in turn increases constipation.

Triphala is a good choice for chronic constipation. Triphala can be given in the dose of 1 to 3 grams at night, with warm water. Triphala has a laxative effect and is made of equal parts of amla, haritaki and bibhitaki. If the triphala causes griping pain when taken (sharp pains in the stomach area) add amla to the triphala in the proportion 1 part amla to 3 parts triphala. Triphala also acts as a rejuvenating medicine for the colon. Ahayarishta is another good medicine for this condition, 30 ml. twice day for 1 month.

Massage

Regular massage to the abdomen and back with the use of proper oils is an excellent treatment for chronic constipation. The patient should be massaged on an empty stomach after their bladder and bowel has been emptied. First apply ample oil over the abdomen. Then use a friction type massage beginning at the lower right side (ileocecal junction), then moving up, across, then downwards following the large intestine. This should be followed by kneading movements which are light at first, and then become deeper and firmer. Later on give a light massage to the back.

Chronic constipation is many times due to a lack of tone in the musculature of the abdominal muscles. This type of massage strengthens the muscles of the abdomen and brings a good tone to the musculature of the colon.

Diet

Correction of dietary habits is a must. It is advisable to eat a lot of green vegetables, plenty of fruit, oily foods and bulk forming foods containing high amounts of roughage or fiber. Food must be taken at the proper time. Irregular food habits can cause constipation.

Gout

According to Ayurveda, vitiated (abnormal) Vata and aggravated blood (rakta) causes this disease, which is referred to as Vatarakta. Increased blood uric acid levels are also responsible for this disease.

Symptoms

Usually the disease starts with inflammation of the big toe or thumb. Following inflammation of the toe or thumb, the other big or small joints in the body are affected. The disease originates in the circulatory system, gets localized into the joints and then spreads throughout the body. The swollen joints are very painful, tender, inflamed, red and warm to the touch. A high degree fever is usually present in the acute stage. Often skin rashes and allergic symptoms are also present with severe itching or a change in the color of the skin. Excessive sweating, or sometimes absence of sweating, and severe pain in the bones and muscles may be present.

Treatment

Purification by medicated purgation or blood letting according to the condition and stage of the disease is advised. Internally, three specific herbs are used. Guduchi (tinospora cordifolia), kokilaksha (astercantha longifolia) or suranjana (colchium luteum) may be taken in the dosage of 1 gram per day of any one of these three herbs.

Massage

Lightly apply oil prepared from guduchi or pinda taila to the swollen joints. Pinda taila is prepared from bees wax, a decoction of majista (rubia cordifolia) and sesame oil. In this condition avoid deep massage. Internally, medicated ghee with guduchi is indicated. A simple combination of 500 mg each of guggulu with guduchi or colchium, twice a day for one month is very useful.

Technique

Depending on the joint involved the masseur should perform a circular massage around the joint.

Headache

Pain anywhere in the body is usually due to Vata vitiation. However, Pitta and Kapha can be also be associated with Vata in the case of headaches. In Ayurveda, headache is classified under the term "Shiro roga". Ayurveda describes 11 types of headaches and other diseases in which headache is the prominent symptom. There are two main causes of headaches, intracranial and extracranial.

Intracranial causes

Trauma, vascular headache due to migraine, hypertension, vasodilator drugs, alcohol hangover, withdrawal of habit forming drugs and caffeine.

Extracranial causes

Trauma to soft tissues of the scalp, bones, and sinuses. Reflex causes from the eyes, ears and teeth also can cause headaches. Similarly stress and strain are responsible for tension headaches.

Symptoms

Vata type headaches are characterized by severe pain with anxiety, constipation, lack of sleep, and depression. It can be due to worry and strain.

Pitta type headaches are accompanied with a burning sensation, pain in the eyes, irritability and photophobia. Migraine headache with nausea, vomiting, blurring of vision, and headaches restricted to one side of the head is usually a Pitta type

Kapha types are a dull, aching pain with cold or heaviness in the head.

In addition to Vata, Pitta and Kapha types there are the following.

Ardhavabhedaka is a typical migraine headache.

Suryavarta - In this type the intensity of the headache increases as the sun rises This is more common in a Pitta type constitution.

Shankhaka - The headache is more prominent in the temporal region.

Anantavata - Due to the vitiation of all doshas. This is a type in which the intensity is very severe.

Massage

Vata type - Apply nimbpatradi oil to the head.

Pitta type - Massage the head with bhringamalakadi oil, padmakadi oil, himasagar oil, amalakyadi oil or neeli bhrungaradi oil.

For all other types of headache use dhanvantara oil, manjishthadi oil, triphaladi oil or durvadi oil is indicated (durva is very thin grass which is similar to Bermuda grass in the west).

Technique

The masseur should pour oil into their palm. They should then dip their fingers in the oil and begin massaging the scalp.

Heart Disease

In Ayurveda, heart disease can be classified due to Vata, Pitta or Kapha. Vata type heart disease includes irregular heartbeats, arrhythmia or pain (angina pectoris). Pitta type heart disease includes inflammatory type diseases such as pericarditis or S.B.E. (subacute bacterial endocarditic). Kapha type heart disease includes congestive heart failure or cardiac asthma.

For Vata type heart disease, Hrid Basti is very effective. Hrid basti is a procedure in which a ring of dough is placed around the heart area which is then filled with oil that has been warmed to body temperature. Narayan oil, chandan bala lakshadi oil or dhanvantara oil should be used for Vata, Pitta or Kapha conditions of the heart. The oil is left in place for 45 minutes. Every 10 to 15 minutes during the procedure some of the oil is removed and replaced with additional warmed oil.

Hemiplegia

Paralysis of one side of the body is known as hemiplegia. In Ayurveda it is called "Pakshavadha." Paksha is hand, foot or one side of the body. Vadha is complete loss of function. It is classified under vatavyadhi (diseases of Vata). Other diseases like paraplegia or facial paralysis (ardita) are also grouped under the category of vatavyadhi.

Causative factors

This is a Vata disorder involving the central nervous system and the muscular system. It can be due to cerebral tumors, embolism or hemorrhage. Other diseases of the brain or head trauma can produce hemiplegia in which there may be paralysis on one side of the body, with or without aphasia (a disorder of speech generation due to a specific brain disease). Prana and vyana subtypes of Vata are vitiated (abnormal) in this disorder.

Treatment

In the case of complete paralysis of all the extremities, the patient, for the first few days or weeks will be totally bedridden. In this case, all necessary nursing care must be taken. A waterbed should be provided to avoid bed sores. Daily passive exercises must be given to avoid disuse atrophy of the extremities. In such a condition the patient is bound to become depressed. Those attending him should keep him engaged in reading or watching television.

Nasya

Nasya can be used to treat prana Vata. The main site of prana is the brain, and the nasal passages are directly connected to the brain. Therefore nasya (nasal instillation of substances) is a direct route to the brain, and thus prana. A tonification type of nasya, with sesame oil medicated with Vata relieving herbs should be used.

Massage and Sudation

Daily massage to the paralyzed limbs along with whole body sudation is indicated. Abhyanga can be with simple sesame or almond oil, or medicated oils such as narayan oil, bala oil, dhanvantari oil or karpasasthyadi oil. Oil massage improves the circulation in the muscles and also helps improve the muscular tone. For sudation, herbs such as vitex negundo, holy basil or camphor should be used.

Medicated enema

The main site of Vata is the large intestine. Enemas are the treatment of choice for reducing Vata as these act directly on the main site of Vata. It is advisable to give alternating cleansing enemas followed by oil enemas. For a cleansing type of enema use a decoction of ten roots (dashamoola) and its paste with oil, ghee, honey and rock salt. For an oil enema use plain sesame oil, 60 to 70 cc., or use medicated oils like narayan or bala oil. A plastic syringe can be used for giving the oil enema. Along with the enema treatment Shiro basti and Shirodhara treatments are also very useful.

Obesity

Obesity is the most common metabolic disorder and is one of the oldest documented diseases. In Ayurveda, as early as 100 BC, the Charaka Samhita described this disorder under the title "Medoroga" or diseased state of fat metabolism. According to Charaka, the great Ayurvedic physician, an individual whose increased adipose and muscle tissue makes the hips, abdomen and breasts pendulous and whose vitality is much less than their body size, is obese.

Charaka has stated that obesity causes a reduction of longevity, premature aging, unpleasant odor, excessive sweating, dyspnea (labored or difficult breathing upon mild exertion), excessive hunger and thirst, weakness, loss of vitality, loss of sexual power, and mental confusion.

Causative factors

Obesity is due to factors such as overeating of heavy, sweet and oily foods, lack of exercise and hereditary predisposition. It can also be due to disorders of the pituitary, thyroid, adrenals, gonads, pancreas and hypothalamus.

The cause of obesity in Ayurveda can be explained as a cycle which perpetuates itself. First, an increase in food intake, due to excess appetite, produces excess Kapha and ama (toxins). This results in a low tissue fire in the fat tissue and thus an excess production of fat. The excess fat then blocks the channels of the body which results in an increase in Vata. One of the main causes of increased Vata is obstruction in the channels (the other main cause of increased Vata is weight loss). Typically when Vata is increased we see a decrease in appetite. However, in the case of obesity we see an exception to this general rule and there is an increase in appetite. With an increase of appetite we have an increase of food intake, and the cycle continues.

Treatment

The Ayurvedic approach to treating obesity is to intervene at all the causative steps, therefore breaking the cycle. Formation of excess Kapha and toxins (ama) is treated by toxin burning herbs such as powdered ginger or trikatu. Trikatu consists of equal parts of black pepper, long pepper and powdered ginger. Later, for detoxification of ama, bitter herbs are used. To increase the tissue fire of the fatty tissue, herbs such as guggulu, carthamus tinctoris, careya arborea and shilajit are used. The channels which have become blocked are treated with herbs like chitraka or barberry, which have a scraping action that opens the channels. Aggravation of Vata is treated by medicated enemas of the cleansing type using decoctions such as dashamula.

Externally, massage is given with herb powders such as calamus (acorus calamus). Mentally, the patient is advised to meditate for increased will power so they can resist those foods which produce both Kapha and ama (see diet below). Regular daily exercise until there is perspiration on the forehead and in the armpit is a must. It can be in the form of cycling, swimming, jogging, running or other outdoor activities.

Massage

Only an udvartana massage (dry powder massage) using dry and hot powders of vacha (acorus calamus) or satala should be used. The massage must be very deep and a little pain producing. Only this type of massage will be able to break up and move the fatty tissue from the thighs, buttocks and other regions.

Diet

Avoid all fried and heavy foods, chocolates, sweets, butter, cheese, paneer (farmers cheese) and meat as well as cold drinks and preserved foods. A light and dry diet is recommended to provide only the necessary energy.

Poliomyelitis

In Ayurveda poliomyelitis has been described as "Bala pakshvadha." It is a Pitta /Vata disease caused by an acute viral infection which affects various parts of the central nervous and muscular systems. It usually affects children under the age of 5 years. However, during epidemics older children and adults can be affected.

Symptoms

In the early stage (prodromal) there may be symptoms of respiratory and gastrointestinal disturbances such as coryza (head cold), sore throat, cough, nausea, vomiting, diarrhea and other symptoms like fever, headache and irritability. These symptoms are more aggravated in the preparalytic stage.

In the paralytic stage, which starts between the second and fifth day, the lower limbs are frequently affected. Rarely is there upper limb paralysis or respiratory disturbance.

Massage

To pacify vitiated (abnormal) Vata external massage is the best treatment. It should be started only when the tenderness in the muscles disappears.

Chandan bala lakshadi oil, narayan oil, mahanarayan oil, dhanvantari oil, bala oil or ksheera bala oil should be gently massaged followed by a warm bath. 100 times fortified ksheera bala oil can be used for internal consumption in a dose of 5 drops twice a day.

Pizhichil, which is pouring hot medicated oil by the drip method on the body is useful. Navarakkizi is another treatment in which the patient is massaged with a rice bolus cooked in medicated milk.

These treatments are often combined with alternate oil enemas and cleansing enemas. Herbs for the cleansing enemas are selected according to the predominance of doshas. Tonifying enemas include mixtures of milk, meat soup, honey, ghee and a decoction of tonifying herbs. The tonifying enema should be given very slowly by a drip method so that the liquid is retained in the body. This type of enema has a beneficial effect of increasing the tone of the paralyzed muscles.

Diet

An anti Vata diet should be given. Plenty of dairy such as milk and ghee should be taken. Meat broth, basmati rice and plenty of green vegetables should also be given.

Rickets

This is a disease occurring in infancy and early childhood due to deficiency of Vitamin D affecting the bones in the body. In Ayurveda it is called "Phakka" and is a Vata disease.

Symptoms

Marasmic children, which are infants who are severely underweight, are seldom rachitic. However, as soon as the infant begins to put on weight rickets is likely to develop. This is because rickets develops only when growth starts taking place and there is a deficiency of Vitamin D and calcium. The infant with rickets is characteristically restless, cries frequently and may perspire excessively. Muscles of the limbs and abdomen become very weak and without tone, with abdominal distention. Normal developmental activities like crawling and sitting are delayed and the eruption of teeth is prolonged. Various deformities in the bones of the skull and thorax develop. The bony deformity may become permanent if it is not treated in time. The treatment should be started as early as possible.

Massage

Regularly massage the baby with any of the following oils. Chandan bala lakshadi oil, dashapak baladi oil, ashwangadhadi oil or narayan oil. In addition to massage, expose the child to early morning sun, or to infra red light, for 15 to 20 minutes daily for one month.

Sciatica

Pain along the distribution of the sciatic nerve due to inflammation is a typical disorder of Vata vitiation. Most often this is due to a lumbar disc prolapse. It can also be due to injury, trauma to the vertebral column or to the nerve proper, various tumors of the spinal cord, or different diseases of the vertebral column such as arthritis, tuberculosis, spondylolisthesis or cancer. Some disorders of the hip joint like fibrositis and some particular disorders of the pelvis also cause this syndrome.

Symptoms

There is severe pain along the root of the sciatic nerve that may travel down the back of the leg to the knee. The patient has difficulty while walking. If the pain is constant, insomnia may also be present.

Treatment

Herbs like ricinus communis, rasna, bala, ashwagandha, guggulu and dashmoola are useful. Cleansing enemas with dashmoola decoction, alternating with oil enemas are indicated.

Kati basti

Kati basti is a special type of basti which is effective in treating this disease It is performed on the back from where the sciatic nerve originates. It is useful in relieving the pain and inflammation. For Kati basti, ask the patient to lie on the abdomen. Prepare a wheat flour dough and make a dam with the dough in a four inch circle over the sciatic area on the back which is inflamed and painful. These wheat flour dams should be able to hold warm medicated oil without leaking. Dhanvantara, bala or narayan oil can be used. Pour the oil into the flour dough dam and leave the oil for 20 minutes.

Massage

In sama (with ama) conditions use vishagarbha or prassarani oil. In nirama (without ama) conditions use Mahanarayana oil. The massage should be done along the line of sciatic nerve.

Massage with vishgarbha oil, saindhavadi oil or prasarini oil is advised. Afterwards, fomentation with holy basil (tulsi) leaves mixed in water using a pressure cooker with a hose attached and directed at the site of pain is very useful.

Sports Massage

Professional sportsmen value massage very highly because it works on several levels Used before exercise it can prepare the body for the increased activity, not only by warming and loosening the muscles and joints, but also by increasing flexibility and helping to prevent cramps and injury. It also stimulates the system both physically and mentally. This is a key to improved performance. After an exercise session, massage speeds up the elimination of waste products by stimulating the lymphatic system. Massage is done for longer periods to the joints than the muscles.

Strain and Sprain

A burning sensation under the skin indicates that the muscle fibers or ligaments have been strained, stretched beyond their natural limit. A routine of pre-exercise massage and limbering will help to prevent strains. Gently massaging the affected area helps speedy recovery.

Sprains are more serious and are caused by violent wrenching of joints, most commonly ankles, wrists or knees. The surrounding muscles, ligaments and tendons may also be damaged and the affected areas may be swollen or painful. Apply ice packs for 15 to 20 minutes. Give a gentle massage to the affected area. The best oils for massage in this condition are prasarani and vishagarbha oil. Similarly, products like myostal liniment or wintergreen oil are also very useful in these conditions

Cramps

Frequent cramps may indicate generally poor circulation. Massage will increase the blood circulation to alleviate the pain.

Varicose veins

Varicose veins are a condition where the veins become distended and knotted. This is primarily a cosmetic problem in women.

Causative factors

Defective or weak valves associated with postural strain, which obstructs venous blood flow, is the main causative factor. Other factors include constipation, irregularity and jobs with continuous standing. They can also be due to pressure in the abdominal cavity from pregnancy. In pregnancy, the varicosity is temporary. In the early stage of varicose veins the patient often consults the doctor for cosmetic purposes only. In later stages, when the varicosity increases, there is pain after standing and the affected leg feels heavy. Vata constitution people suffer most from this disorder.

Treatment

It is important that the patient not wear tight clothing which constricts the circulation. Ask the patient to apply elastic bandages at the affected area of the leg to prevent further development of varicosity. For women, wearing any type of stockings that provide support helps in prevention. It is also advisable to raise the legs while sleeping at least for 1 to 2 hours every day.

Massage

Never carry out a kneading type of massage or put pressure on the varicose veins. Use warm sesame oil, narayan oil or bala oil in an upward direction, from foot to groin, twice a day. After massage keep the leg in warm water for fomentation. This will strengthen the valves in the veins and the condition will improve.

CHAPTER 14

HEALING SYSTEMS RELATED TO MASSAGE

Traditional Chinese Medicine (TCM)

Ayurveda and Traditional Chinese Medicine (TCM) may be the two oldest healing system still practiced widely today. Both Ayurveda and TCM believe in maintaining the equilibrium of energies in the body, and both talk about the importance of the five basic elements. Traditional Chinese Medicine places a focus on balancing the yin and yang energies in the body and tries to maintain their equilibrium with herbs, diet, acupuncture and body work. TCM believes that energy flows through certain meridians, and blockage can cause disturbance or diseases in the body. To relieve this blockage acupuncture and acupressure is helpful.

Reflexology

It is said that early Egyptian and Chinese civilizations were practicing this science which is sometimes called "Zone Therapy". The basis of this therapy is that reflex zones on the hands and feet are related to different organs and systems of the body. These organs and systems can be stimulated for health and therapeutic purposes through massage and manipulation of the hands and feet. Reflexology states that the body can be divided into ten vertical zones, each corresponding to an area of the hand or foot, so that the hands and feet are in effect a map of the body. A sensitive area of the hand or foot indicates a problem in the corresponding organ or system of the body and by working on the appropriate painful spot the problem can be solved.

Use of proper oils and manipulation on these areas can bring about,
- Reduction of stress and strain
- Stimulation of different organs, systems and glands for health promotion as well as for treatment purposes
- Removal of obstructions in the channels allowing a free flow of energy throughout the body for revitalizing energy levels and maintaining equilibrium

Technique

Hold one foot with both your hands. Begin with some relaxing movements like ankle rotation and ankle stretch. Stroke the foot softly from the ankles to the toes to smooth and relax the whole area of the foot. Use techniques like thumb hooking, thumb walking and finger walking. Find the sore spots on the sole of the foot. Select a proper oil and massage these points slowly.

Shiatsu

Although the roots of this system can be traced to ancient Chinese medicine it is a modern Japanese therapy. The word 'shi' means finger and 'atsu' means pressure. This is now recognized in Japan as a traditional system along with Japanese massage (Asuma).

Shiatsu is a manipulative therapy which uses pressure applied to specific points and meridian lines all over the body. Practitioners of this system use their thumbs, elbows, knees and heels along the entire network of pressure points and meridian lines. The main aim of this pressure is to balance the energies in the body, known as Qi or Ki, to prevent disease and maintain health. With knowledge of the pressure points a Shiatsu expert can diagnose and treat any condition in which there is an imbalance in the body energies.

There are 660 zones where vessels, glands and nerves come together. These zones are called "tsubo". Although they are invisible on the skin, experts can locate them. The Hara is considered one of the most powerful energy centers of the body. It is located in the abdominal area. An experienced therapist can diagnose imbalances in the organs and meridians by observing the flow of Qi in the Hara.

An important principle of this type of massage is to have simultaneous touch from both hands. With a two hand connection, a circuit can be established. One hand is kept stationary while the other hand moves.

Shiatsu is known to have a calming influence on hypertension, while increasing blood pressure when it is too low. Many people also find this to be a good technique for relieving pain and stress.

Technique

There are two main techniques, namely palming and thumbing. In palming the palms are placed on the body of the patient to establish contact and used to exert different pressures on the body. In thumbing, pressure is given using the thumbs.

Chiropractic

Daniel David Palmer invented this method of healing. This science believes that most of our physical problems are related with misaligned or subluxed vertebrae and that with proper alignment these problems can be treated. Alignment used by chiropractors is essentially the same as that of osteopaths, with chiropractors restricting it to the spine while osteopaths work on any affected joint, even the relatively immobile joints of the cranium.

Osteopathy

This is also referred to as "bone treatment". It is an invention of Andrew Taylor who was a Swedish allopathic doctor.

Silk Glove Massage

Massage with raw silk gloves is good for kapha constitution types. The gloves are coarse and rough and provide both increased friction and pressure allowing for a deeper massage.

Chromassi

This is a system based on Chrono-massage, which is used for painful syndromes and chronic diseases. This is a combination of massage and acupressure. Available computer software for this system can be used for teaching and clinics and is available from the Institute of Computer Science, Academy of Sciences, Prague, Czech Republic.

Massage with Instruments

There are many electrical instruments which have a vibratory action, as well as simple wooden rollers which can be used for massage. These instruments have a very limited use compared to the different massage strokes, medicinal oils and powders which can be utilized.

CHAPTER 15

RESEARCH ON MASSAGE

All over the world various medical institutes have performed research on the effects of massage in relation to the physiology of the body as well as the effect of massage in treating different diseases.

The Medical Library at Bethesda, Maryland , USA, has collected this research data. This research is available in India from the National Informatic Center, Pune, in the "Medlars and Gistnic Database" section. The information available contains over 600 pages. The following is a listing of some of the research available in the database.

Stress and Strain

The effect of brief massage therapy, music therapy and visual imagery on muscle relaxation at a major public hospital. The effects were assessed using a pre/post test design in 100 employees. Result showed that the therapies, when applied for short periods of time, are equally effective for reducing stress among hospital employees. University of Miami School of Medicine, Florida, 33101, USA

Aromatherapy and Massage for Geriatric Care

The appropriate use of these therapies is useful in conventional treatment regimens Associate degree Nursing program, Ohio University of Zenesville, USA.

Headache

Foot reflex zone massage was found effective. Institute for Pflegeforschung, Bern, Germany.

Use of Massage in Sports Medicine

Massage is beneficial to increase blood flow, healing of connective tissues and edema. School of Occupational Therapy and Physiotherapy, University of East Angelia, Norwich, UK.

Peptic Ulcer and GI Tract Diseases

Compared to conventional treatment, deep reflex muscular massage for treatment of peptic ulcer patients, shows positive changes in adaptive compensatory systems.

Tension Headaches

81 patients were treated with massage, vibration etc. Excellent results were obtained at JFK medical center, Wellington regional medical center, Atlantis, Florida, USA.

Pressure Sores

Regular massage of the bony prominance can prevent bedsores. Maastritcht Uniersity, Faculty of Health Sciences, Department of Nursing science, Nedarlands.

Cerebral Circulatory Disorders

119 patients who have suffered an episode of reversible brain ischaemia were studied in this project to find out the effect of massage of different areas of the body on the cerebral hemodynamics.

Job stress

Short massage therapy produced immediate relief in hospital workers. University of Miami, USA.

Asthma

32 children with asthma were randomly assigned to receive massage or relaxation therapy. The younger children who received massage showed immediate decrease in behavioral anxiety and improved pulmonary functions. Touch Research Institute, University of Miami, USA.

Chronic Low Backache

Relaxation, corrective manual modulation and improving postural drawbacks produced great relief. Christie Clinic Association, Dept. of Sports Medicine, Rantoul, IL, 61866 USA

Cancer Pain

Development of massage service to cancer patients as complimentary therapy is useful in reducing many problems. Radiotherapy department, Hammersmith hospital, London, UK. and Northwestern Ontario Regional Cancer Center, Canada

Pregnancy

26 pregnant women were assigned to massage therapy for 5 weeks. This produced reduction in anxiety, improved mood, better sleep and less back

pain. Touch Research Institute, Florida, USA.

Sleep Disturbance

Critically ill patients are deprived of sleep and its healing qualities. 69 patients were randomly selected and were given 6 minute back massage along with a 6 minute relaxation technique. It was found that back massage was useful for promoting sleep University of Arkansas, College of Nursing, Little Rock, USA.

Post Mastectomy Lymphoedema and Massage

Multi model therapy reduced lymphodematous limb volume in 18 out of 25 patients. Wesley Clinic for Hematology and Oncology.

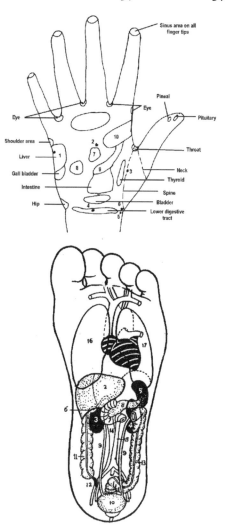

APPENDIX 1

MEDICATED AND AROMATIC (ESSENTIAL) OILS

Preparation of Medicated Oils

Usually 1 part of the paste (kalka) of the herbs is mixed with 4 parts of oil and 16 parts of liquid . The liquid can be the juice of the herbs, a decoction, milk, etc. The liquid and the paste (kalka) are mixed together and then the oil is added. The mixture is boiled, stirring continuously so that the paste does not adhere to the bottom of the pan. From time to time some paste is taken out of the vessel and its condition is tested. The medicated oil has three stages of cooking or paka.

1. Mrudu paka

   In this stage the paste remaining at the bottom of the pan can be rolled between the fingers without sticking and is waxy in nature. When a cotton wick is dipped in this paste and lit on fire this paste will burn with a slight crackling sound as it still contains some water.

2. Madhyama paka

   When the mixture is boiled further the paste becomes harder. A cotton wick, when dipped in the paste and lit on fire, burns without any crackling sound indicating that the water has been evaporated. The oil prepared up to this stage is used for nasya and for external purposes.

3. Khara paka

   When further heat is given to the mixture the oil has a typical smell, color and texture. At this stage the paste begins to fry in the oil. This oil can be used for abhyanga and for basti.

Important Oil Preparations

Agaru oil - Agaru, bilva, yashtimadhu and sesame oil (BR).

Amalaki oil - Amalaki, haritaki, bibhitaka, bilva, sariva, ela and sesame oil (BR).

Amruta oil - Tinispora cordifolia, triphala and sesame oil (BR).

Arjuna oil - Decoction of the bark of arjuna and sesame oil (YR).

Asana-bilvadi oil - Asana, bilva, bala, amruta, licorice, triphala, milk, coconut oil (SY).

Asana eladi oil - Asana, ela, jeevanti, bilva, bala roots, deodara, sesame oil (SY).

Ashwagandhadi oil - Ashwagandha and sesame oil (BR).

Bala oil - Bala, guduchi, rasna, ela, agaru, manjishtha, atibala, licorice, tulsi, lavanga, kankola, nafgakeshara and sesame oil (AH).

Bilvadi oil - Bilva, goat milk and sesame oil (SS).

Brahmi oil - Brahmi and coconut oil (YR).

Brihat Saindhavadi oil - Rock salt (saindhava), arka, maricha, chitraka, haridra and sesame oil (BR).

Bhrungamalakadi oil - Juice of bhringaraja and amalaka, licorice, milk and sesame oil (SY).

Bhrungaraja oil - Eclipta alba, manjishtha, lodhra, bala, daruharidra, licorice, sandalwood, and sesame oil (BR).

Chandanadi oil - Santalum album, licorice, vetivera zizanoides, jatamansi, agaru, bala, bilwa, kutki, sesame oil (YR).

Chandan-bala-lakshadi oil - Red and white sandalwood, bala root, laksha, madhuka, deodaru, manjishtha, agaru, ashwagandha, rasna, katuki, and sesame oil (YR).

Dashamuladi oil- Dashamula and sesame oil (YR).

Dashamula is a collection of ten different roots which includes
1. shaliparni (desmodium gangeticum),
2. prushniparni (uraria picta),
3. bruhati (solanum xanthocarpum)
4. bruhati (solanum solanum indicum),
5. gokshura (tribulus terestris),
6. bilwa (aegle marmelos),
7. shyonaka (oroxylum indicum),

8. patala (sterospermum suaveolens),
9. agnimanth (premna integrifolia),
10. kashamari (gmelina arboria),

Devadarvyadi oil - Devadaru and sesame oil (YR).

Dhanvantara oil - Bala roots, cow's milk, kushtha, bilva, patala, agaru, sandalwood, vacha, punarnava, licorice, sariva, haritaki, amalaki, (AH and Vaidya Yogaratnavali).

Doorvadi oil - Durva, nimba, narikala ksheera, licorice and coconut oil (AH).

Gandha oil - Herbs in the kakolyadi group (kakoli, kshira kakoli, black gram, medha, mahameda, guduchi, jeevanti, kakadshingi, vanshal-ochana, cow's milk and sesame oil (AH).

Himasagara oil - Shatavari, kushmanda, vidari, tagara, chandana, man-jishtha, agaru, licorice, lodhra, musta, shalmali and sesame oil (BR).

Jeerakadi oil - Jeeraka and sesame oil (YR).

Jyotishmati oil - Jyotishmati, apamargaand apamarga (YR).

Karpas-asthyadi oil - Karpasa seeds, bala, masha, kullatha, sarshapa, ras-na, deodaru, punarnava, shigru, kushtha, milk of goat and coconut oil (SY).

Kshara oil - Plant alkali of apamarga, vacha, shunthi, kushtha, deodaru and sesame oil (BR)

Kshirabala oil - Bala roots, decoction of bala, cow's milk and sesame oil (AH).

Kottamachukadi oil - Kushtha, musta, acorus calamus, garlic, deodaru, sarshapa, curds and sesame oil (SY).

Kumkumadi oil - Kumkum, ushira, laksha, chandana, yashtimadhu, na-gakeshara, manjishtha, teja patra, padmaka, kushtha, gorochana, laksha, daruharidra, priyangu, vacha and sesame oil (YR).

Lakshadi oil - Laksha, haridra, manjishtha, rasna, ashwagandha and ses-ame oil (BR).

Lashunadi oil - Garlic pulp, juice and sesame oil (CD).

Mahamasha oil - Masha, dashamula, vacha, maricha, gokshura and sesame oil (BR).

Maha manjishthadi oil - Manjishtha, bilva, agnimantha, patala, bruhati, bala, rasna, ashwagandha, punarnava, atibala, sandalwood, manjishtha, kushtha, ela, musta, camphor, sesame oil (BR).

Mahanarayan oil - Bilva, ashwagandha, bruhati, gokshura,, bala, kantakari, atibala, rasna, deodaru, agaru, haritaki, ela, licorice, vacha, sesame oil (BR).

Manjishthadi oil - Manjishtha, sariva, musta, katuka, jatiphala, triphala, kushtha, jatamansi, juice of kumari and sesame oil (SY).

Masha oil - Masha and sesame oil (BR).

Nalapamaradi oil - Juice of fresh curcuma, parpata, udumbara, plaksha, triphala, agaru, kushtha, and sesame oil (SY).

Narayan oil - Shatavari, dashamula, punarnava, ashwagandha, kantakari, jatamansi, vacha, kushtha, milk and sesame oil (BR).

Nimba oil - Juice of leaves of nimba and sesame oil (BR).

Nimba patradi oil - Juice of leaves of nimba, eclipta alba, shatavari, manjishtha, licorice, ushira, musta, amruta, sariva, milk and sesame oil (SY).

Nirgundi oil (shefali oil) - Juice of nirgundi and sesame oil.

Padmakadi oil - Lotus stem, doorva, sesame oil (BR).

Pinda oil - Bees wax, manjishtha, sarjarasa, sariva, dhanyamla, and sesame oil (AH).

Sahachara oil - Sahachara, bilva, gokshura, chandana, shilajita, and sesame oil (AH).

Shankhapushpi oil - Shankhapushpi, bilva, agaru and sesame oil (YR).

Triphaladi oil - Triphala, guduchi, bala, eranda, kushtha, ushira, musta, milk, sesame oil (SY).

Vacha oil - Vacha, haritaki, laksha, kutaki and sesame oil (AH).

Vacha lashunadi oil - Vacha, lashuna and sesame oil (SY).

Vishagarbha oil - Datura alba, kushtha, vatsanabha, vacha, chitraka and sesame oil (YR).

Vrushchika oil - Boil sesame oil and put a live scorpion into the oil. Keep the oil boiling for 5 minutes and then remove the scorpion. This is one of the best oils for external use for relieving pain anywhere in the body.

Aromatic or Essential Oils

Basil - Ocimum sanctum
Bay - Pimenta racemosa
Benzoin - Stryax benzoin
Bergamot - Citrus bergania
Cedar wood - Juniperus virginiana
Chamomile - Anthemis nobilis
Cinnamon - Cinnamomum zeylanicum
Comfrey - Symphtum offiicnale
Cypress - Cupressus sempervirens
Eucalyptus - Eucalyptus globulus
Fennel - Foeniculum vulgare
Frankincense - Boswellia thurifera
Geranium - Pelargonium adorantissimum
Hyssop - Hyssopus officinalis
Jasmine - Jasminum officinale
Juniper - Juniperus communis
Lavender - Lavendula officinalis
Lemon - Citrus limonum
Lemongrass - Cymbopogon citratus
Marjoram - Origanum marjorana
Melissa - Melisa officinalis
Myrrh - Comiphora myrrh
Neroli - Citrus aurantium
Orange - Citrus aurantium or sinesis
Parsley - Petroselinum sativum
Patchouli - Pogostemon patchouli
Peppermint - Mentha piperata
Pine - Pinus sylvestris
Rose - Rosa centigolia
Rosemary - Rosamarinus officinalis
Sage - Salvia officinalis
Sandalwood - Santalum album
Tea Tree - Melaleuca alternifolia
Thyme - Thymus vulgaris
Ylang Ylang- Cananga odorata

APPENDIX 2

INDEX OF BOTANICAL HERBS

SANSKRIT	ENGLISH	BOTANICAL NAME
Abhaya	Myrobalan	Terminalia chebula
Agaru	Eaglewood	Aquilaria agallocha
Agasti	Agati	Sesbania grandiflora
Agnimantha	Clerodendrum	Phlomidis
Agnimantha	-	Premna integrifolia
Ahiphena	Opium	Papaver somniferum
Ajagandha	-	Gynandropsis pentaphylla
Ajamoda	Celery seed	Carum ajmoda / roxburghianum
Akarakarabha	Pellitory roots	Anacyclus pyrethrum
Akshotaka	Wall Nut	Juglans regia
Amalaki	-	Emblica officinalis
Amaravel	Doddar	Cuscuta reflaxa
Amlavetasa	-	Garcinia pedunculata
Amlavetasa	Sorrel	Rumex vesicarius
Amra	Mango	Magnifera indica
Amragandhi haridra	-	Curcuma amada
Amruta	-	Tinospora cordifolia
Ananta	-	Hemidesmus sarsaparela indicus
Apamarga	Rough chapp tree	Achyranthes aspera
Aparajita	Butterfly pea	Clitoria ternatea
Aragvadha	-	Casia fistula
Arishtaka	Soap nut	Sapindus trifoliatus
Arjuna	-	Terminalia arjuna
Asana	-	Pterocarpus marsupium
Ashoka	Ashok Tree	Saraca indica
Ashvagol	-	Plantago ovata
Ashwagandha	Winter cherry	Withania somniferous
Ashwattha	-	Ficus religiosa
Asthisandhanaka	-	Cissus quadrangularis
Atasi	Linseed	Linum usitatissimum
Atibala	Indian Mellow	Abutilon indicum
Ativisha	Indian Attees	Aconitum heterophyllum
Avartaki	Tanners Cassia	Cassia auriculata
Avartani	Indian Screw tree	Helicteres isora
Babbula	Indian Gum Tree	Acacia
Bakuchi	Bavachi	Psoralea corylifolia

Bakula	Indian Medler	Mimusops elengi
Bala	-	Sida cordifolia
Banapsha	-	Viola odorata
Bhallataka	Marking Nut	Semicarpus anacardium
Bhanga	Marijuana	Cannabis sativa
Bhringaraja	-	Eclipta alba
Bibhitaka	-	Terminalia chebula
Bilva	Bael	Aegle marmelos
Bola	-	Commiphora myrrh
Brahmi	Indian Pennywort	Bacopa moniera
Bruhati	Indian Nightshade	Solanum indicum
Chakramarda	-	Cassia tora
Champaka	-	Michelia champaka
Chandana	Sandalwood	Santalum album
Chandrashura	Watercress	Lepidium sativum
Changeri	-	Oxalis corniculata
Chavika / Chavya	-	Piper chaba
Chincha	-	Plumbago rosea
Chitraka	Leadwort	Plumbago zeylanica
Chopachini	China root	Smilax china
Dadima	Pomegranate	Punica granatum
Danti	-	Baliospermum mortanum
Danti	Wild croton	Croton polyandrum
Daruharidra	Indian barberies	Barberis aristata
Davana	-	Artemissia palenf
Devdaru	Doddar	Cedrus deodara
Dhanyaka	Coriander	Coriandrum sativum
Dhataki	Fulsee flower	Woodfordia fruticosa
Dhatriphala	-	Barringtonia acutangula
Dhatura Krishna	Thorn apple	Datura metal
Dhatura shweta	Thorn apple	Datura stramonium
Draksha	Grape	Vitis vinifera
Dronapushpi	-	Leucas cephalotes
Duralabha	-	Fagonia cretica
Dhanvayasa	-	Alhagi pseudalhagi
Durva	Creeping cyndon	Cyndon dactylon
Ela	cardamom	Elettaria cardamomum
Erandkarkati	Papaya tree	Carica papaya
Erandmool	Castor oil tree	Ricinus communis
Falgu	Fig Tree	Ficus carica
Gajapippali	Elephant piper	Scindapsus officinalis
Gambhari	White teak	Gmelina arborea
Gandha shathi	-	Hedychium spicatum

Gangeruki	-	Canthium parviflorum
Garjar	Carrot	Daucus carota
Gojivha	-	Onosma bracteatum
Gokshura	Calitrops	Tribulus terrestris
Guduchi	-	Tinospora cordifolia
Guggul	-	Balsamodendron mukul
Gunja	Bead Tree	Abrus precatorius
Hamspadi	Maidan hair	Adiantum lunulatum
Hapuspha	Juniper	Juniperus communis
Haridra	Turmeric	Curcuma longa
Hasishudha	-	Heliotropium indicum
Hingu	Assafoetida	Ferula assafoetida
Hingupatri	White emetic nut	Peucedanum grande
Hriber	-	Pavonia deodorata
Ikshu	Sugarcane	Saccharum officinarum
Indravaruni Colocynth,	Citrullus bitter apple	colocynthis
Indrayawa	Kurchi	Holerrhena antidysenterica
Ingudi Zacum	Oil plant	Balanites ingudi
Irimeda	-	Acacia farnesiana / leucopholea
Isabgol	Spogel	Plantago ovata
Ishvari	Indian birchwort	Aristolchia indica
Jaiphala	Croton seed	Croton tiglium
Jambira	Lemon	Citrus medica
Jambu	Black plum	Eugenia jambolana
Jatamasi	Musk root	Nardostachys jatamasi
Jatipatri	Mace	Myristica fragrans
Jatiphal	Nutmeg	Myristica fragrans
Jiraka	Cumin seed	Cuminum cyminum
Jivanti	-	Leptadenia reticulata
Jyotishmati	Stuff tree	Celastrus paniculatus
Kababchini	Cubeb	Piper cubeba
Kadamba	-	Anthocephalus cadamba
Kadali	Banana	Musa sapientum / paradisiaca
Kakajangha	-	Leea acquata
Kakmachi	Black night shade	Solanum nigrum
Kakmari	-	Anamirta cocculus
Kalmegh	Creat	Andrographis paniculata
Kampilla	Kamilla	Mallotus philippinensis
Kanchanara	-	Bauhinia variegata
Kandiari	Jujube fruit	Zinziphus mauuritiana
		Zinziphus phillippinesis
Kantakari	-	Solanum xanthocarpum
Kapikachchu	Cowhage plant	Mucuna pruriens

Kapittha	Wood apple	Feronia elephantum
Karanja	-	Pongomia glabra
Karchura	-	Hedychium spicatum
Karkatashringhi	Galls	Rhus succedanea
Karpas	Indian cotton	Gossypium herbaceum
Karpura	Camphor	Cinnamomum camphora
Karvira	-	Nerium indicum
Kasani	-	Cicorum endiva
Kasmarda	-	Cassia occidentalis
Katphala	Box myrtal	Myrica nagi
Katuka	Hellbore	Picrorhiza kurroa
Ketaki	Keora	Pandanus odoratissim
Khadira	Catechu tree	Acacia catechu
Kharjura	Date palm	Phoenix dactylifera
Kirata Chiretta	-	Swertia chirata
Kirmani	-	Artemisia maritima
Kitmari yavani	-	Aristolchia bracteata
Kokilaksha	-	Asteracantha longifolia
Krushna jiraka	Caraway seeds	Carum carvi
Kuberaksha	Bondu	Caesalpinia bonducella
Kulattha	-	Dolichos biflorus
Kulinjana	Galangal	Alpinia officinarum
Kumari	Aloe	Aloe vera
Kumuda	-	Nymphaea alba
Kunkuma	Saffron	Crocus sativus
Kupilu	-	Strychnus nuxvomica
Kushmanda	-	Benincasa hispida
Kushtha	Costus	Sausurea lappa
Kutaj	Conessi bark	Holarrhena antidysenterica
Lajjalu	Sensitive plant	Mimosa pudica
Laksha	Lac	Cocculus lack
Langali	Superbily	Gloriosa superba
Lashuna	Garlic	Allium sativum
Latakaranja	-	Caesalpinia crista
Lavanga	Clove	Syzygium aromatica
Lodhra	Lodhra	Symplocos recemosa
Lohban	-	Styrax benzoin
Madana	Emetic nut	Randia dumetorum
Madayantika	-	Lawsonia inermis
Madhuka	Mahua tree	Bassia latifolia
Mahanimba	-	Melia azadirachta
Maiphala	-	Quercus infectoria
Majuphala	Gallnut	Quercus infectoria

Mamira	-	Coptis teeta
Mandukaparni	-	Hydrocotyl asiatica
Manjatak	-	Eulophia compestris
Manjistha	Madder root	Rubia cordifolia
Mansala	Guava	Psidium guyava
Maricha (rakta)	Red chili	Capsicum fruitescens
Maricha	Black pepper	Piper nigrum
Markandi	Senna	Cassia angustifolia
Mashaparni		Termanus labialis
Matulunga	Adams apple	Citrus medica
Mendika	Henna	Lawsonia alba
Methika	Fenugreek	Trigonella foenum-graceum
Mnjatak	Salep	Eulophia compestris
Mocharas	-	Bombax malabaricum
Moolaka	Garden radish	Raphanus sativus
Moorva	-	Clematis triloba
Muchkunda	-	Pterospermum indicus
Mudga	-	Phaseolus radiatus
Mundi	-	Sphaeranthus indicus
Musli (black)	-	Curculigo orchioides
Musli	-	Asparagus adscendens
Musta	Nutgrass	Cyperus rotundus
Nadihingu	Gummy gardenia	Gardenia gummifera
Nagarjuni	Australian asthma weed	Euphorbia pilulifera
Nagkeshar	Cobras Saffron	Mesua ferrea
Narikel	Coconut	Cocos nucifera
Nilika	Indigo	Indigofera tinctoria
Nimbuka	Lemon	Citrus acida
Nirgundi	-	Delphinium denudatum
Padma	Lotus	Nelumbium speciosum
Padmaka	Himalayan cherry	Prunus cerasoides
Palandu	Onion	Allium cepa
Palash	Butta	Butea frondosa
Parasika yavani	-	Hyocymus reticulata
Parasika Yavani	Henbane	Hyocymus niger
Paribhadra	Indian coral tree	Erythrina indica
Parijataka	-	Nyctanthus arborstristis
Parnabeeja	-	Kalanchoe pinneta
Pashanabheda	-	Bergenia ligulata
Patanga	Sappan wood	Cacsesalpinia sapan
Patla	Trumpet flower	Stereospermum suaveslens
Patola	Wild Snake	Trichosanthes dioica
Pippala	Sacred Fig	Ficus religiosa

Pippali	Long Pepper	Piper longum
Pippalimoola	Piper longum roots	Piper longum
Pishach Karpas	Abrona	Abroma augusta
Pitta Papara	-	Fumaria officinalis
Priyala	-	Buchanania latifolia
Priyangu	Aglaia	Callicarpa roxburghiana/macrophylla
Prushniparni	-	Uraria logopoides
Pruthvika	-	Nigella sativa
Puga	Betel nut	Areca catechu
Punarnva rakta	Spreading hogwood	Boerhaavia diffusa
Pushkaramula	-	Inula racemosa
Putiha	-	Mentha spicata
Putrajivaka	-	Putranjiva roxburghi
Rakta chandan	Red sandalwood	Pterocarpus santalinus
Rakta niryas	Indian kino tree	Calamus draco
Rasanjana	Barberis	Berberis aristata
Rasna	-	Vanda roxburghii
Revand chini	-	Rheum emodi
Rohitak	-	Ammora rohitak
Rudraksha	-	Elaeocarpus ganitrus
Sahachar	Yellow madar	Barleria prionitis
Sahadevi	-	Vernonia cinerea
Samudra Palak	Elephant creeper	Argyreia speciosa
Saptaparni	Dita	Alstonia scholaris
Saptarangi	-	Caeseria esculanta
Sarala	Long leaf pine	Pinus longifolia / roxburghi
Sariva	-	Hemidesmus indicus
Sarja	-	Vateria indica
Sarpagandha	-	Rauwolfia serpentina
Shal	Yellow resin	Shorea robusta
Shalaparni	Ticktrefoil	Desmodium gangeticum
Shalmali	-	Bombax malabaricum
Shankhapushpi	-	Convolvulus microphyllus
Sharpunkha	Purple tephrosia	Tephrosia purpurea
Shatavari	-	Asparagus racemosus
Shatavha	Dill	Peucedanum graveolens
Shati	Zeodary	Curcuma zedoaria
Shatpushpa	Fennel	Foeniculum vulgare
Shigru	Drumstick tree	Moringa pterygosperma
Shirish	-	Albizzia lebbeck
Shunthi	Ginger root	Zingiber officinalis
Shwet Dhatura	-	Datura alba
Shwet Kanchan	Mountain ebony	Bauhinia recemosa

Shyonaka	-	Oroxylum indicum
Snuhi	-	Euphorbia nerifolia
Somlata	Ephedra	Epherdra vulgaris
Sudarshan	-	Crinum zeylanicum
Suran	-	Amorphophalus companullatus
Surinjan	Colchicum	Colchicum luteum
Suvarnaka	Indian labournam	Cassia fistula
Suvarnakshiri	Yellow thistle	Argemone mexicana
Tagara	Indian valerian	Valeriana wallichii
Talispatra	-	Abies webbina
Tambula	Betel leaf	Piper betel
Tila	Sesame	Sesamum indicum
Tinduka	Ebony	Diospyros embryopteris
Tintidika	Tamarind	Tamarindus indica
Trayanti	Gold thread	Delphinium zalil
Trivruta	Turpeth root	Ipomea turpethum
Tulsi	Holy Basil	Ocimum sanctum
Tuveraka	Chalmogra	Hydnocarpus wightiana
Twak	Cinnamon	Cinnamomum zeylanicum
Udumbara	Fig tree	Ficus glomerata
Ushira	Cuscus grass	Vetiveria zizaniodes
Vacha	Sweet flag	Acorus calmus
Vanharidra	Wild turmeric	Curcuma aromatica
Vanshlochana	Bamboo camphor	Bamboo manna
Varuna	-	Crataeva religiosa
Vasaka	-	Adhatoda vasica
Vata	Banyan Tree	Ficus bengalensis
Vatasnabha	Aconite	Aconitum ferox
Vatghani	Wind killer	Clerodendeum phlomidis
Vidanga	-	Embelia ribes
Vidari	-	Pueraria taberosa
Vijaya	Indian hemp	Cannabis indica
Vijayasara	Indian kino tree	Pterocarpus marsupium
Vishatinduka	Nux vomica	Strychnos nuxvomica
Yashtimadhu	Licorice	Glycerrhiza glabra
Yava	Barly	Hordeum valgare
Yavasaka	Comb thorn	Alhagi camelorum
Yawani	Bishopweed	Carum copticum

APPENDIX 3

SANSKRIT ENGLISH GLOSSARY

Abhighata sahatva - increases immunity to bear trauma
Abhyanga - application of oil to the body
Adhipati - the overlord
Aghata - percussion
Alochaka - sub-type of Pitta, for subtle digestion required for sense organs
Ama - toxin
Amsa - shoulder
Anguli peedana- kneading with cushion of fingers
Anuloma - away from the heart in
Apana - sub-type of Vata, controlling downward movement of feces, urine etc.
Asthi - bone
Asthigata Vata - osteo arthritis
Atharva Veda - type of Veda
Avalambaka - sub- type of kapha, protecting lungs
Avapeedana - light kneading
Ayu - life
Ayu kara - promotes longevity
Ayurveda - Science of life
Basti - bladder
Bhrajaka - sub-type of Pitta, digestion of oils and medicines applied to skin
Bodhaka - sub type of kapha, protecting buccal cavity
Brahmrandra - anterior fontenale
Chavitti - massage with feet
Chedyam- hacking
Dhatu - tissue
Dosha - biological humor
Droni - Traditional wooden table for massage
Drushti prasada kara - beneficial to eyes
Dugdha dhara - drip of milk on head
Gharshana - to rub
Guda - anus
Gulpha - ankle joint
Harshana - vibration
Hridaya - heart
Janu - knee joint
Kampa - vibration

Karna purana - filling the ears with oil
Kesamardana - shampooing the hairs
Kleda - subtle waste product
Kledaka - sub-type of kapha, protecting G I tract
Klesha sahatva - increases strength of the skin to bear pain
Kshipra - quick
Kundalini - serpant power lying dormant at the base of the spine.
Kurcha - knot or bundle of muscles
Lata - veshtana- spiral friction
Mahabharata - Mythological epic
Mala - waste product
Mamsa - facia
Mandhana - muscle rolling
Mardana - massage with friction or pressure
Marma - vital area
Meda - fatty tissue
Mohan - jo-daro - ancient city in India
Nabhi - naval
Nasya - nasal medication
Navarakizi - massage with rice bolus
Netra basti - bathing eye in ghee or oil
Netra tarpana - bathing eye with ghee or oil
Nirama - without toxin
Oleation - application of oils, either internal or external
Pachaka - sub-type of Pitta, for primary digestion of the food
Padaghata - massage with feet
Pari-peedana- Petrissage
Peedana - kneading
Phenaka - producing lather foam
Pichu - cotton pad or towel
Pichu dharana - holding or keeping a cotton towel or pad dipped in oil on
        the head
Pizhichil - massage with warm oil drip
Praharana - percussion
Prakruti - bio-typology, constitution
Prana - sub-type of Vata, controlling inward movement of food, air, water
Pra - peedana - deep kneading
Pratiloma - towards the heart
Pushtikara - nourishes body
Rakta - particulate matter in the blood
Ramayana - Indian mythological epic
Ranjaka - sub-type of Pitta, for secondary digestion
Rasa - plasma

Sadhaka - sub-type of Pitta, for digestion of knowledge
Sama - with ama
Samana - sub type of Vata, controlling movement of food through and the
    secretion of digestive juices in the gastro intestinal tract
Sama prakruti - balanced constitution
Samvahana - massage
Sandhi chalana - movement of joints
Sandhigata Vata - rheumatoid arthritis
Seemanta - the summit, the skull and surrounding joints
Shikha - crest of the skull
Shiro dhara - oil drip on the head
Shiro mardana - head massage
Shleshaka - sub-type of kapha lubricating the joints
Shrama hara - removes fatigue
Shrungataka - place where four roads meet
Shukra - reproductive tissue
Snayu - muscle
Snehana - oleation, lubrication
Sparsha - touch
Sudation (Swedana) - sweating therapy (see swedana)
Sutwak kara - makes skin soft
Swapna kara - gives proper sleep
Swedana - sweating therapy, also known as fomentation
Takra dhara - drip of buttermilk on head
Talahridaya - heart of the palm and sole
Tarpaka - sub-type of kapha, protecting brain
Trasana - stroking
Udana - sub-type of Vata, controlling the outward movement of air
Udgharshana - reinforced friction
Udvartana - massage with dry powders
Udveshtana - wringing
Utsadana - massage with herbal paste
Uzichil - massage with medicated herbs
Vaadyam - tapping
Vata rakta - gouty arthritis
Veda - knowledge
Vitap - perinium
Vyana - sub-type of Vata, controlling movements of the heart and muscles

Classical Textbook Abbreviations

AH -	Ashtanga Hridaya
Ch -	Charaka Samhita
Su -	Sushruta Samhita
BR -	Bhaishajya Ratnavali
SS-	Siddhayoga Sangraha
SY -	Sahasra Yoga
YR -	Yoga Ratnakara

BIBLIOGRAPHY

1. Andrew Weil, Health and Healing, Houghton Mifflin, Boston : 1998.
2. Andrew Weil, Natural Health, Natural Medicine, Houghton Mifflin Company, Boston, USA, 1990
3. Ashtang Hridayam, Varanasi, India, Chaukhamba Krishnadas Academy, reprint 2007
4. Ayurveda, The Gentle Health System, Hans H Rhyner, Motilal Banarasidas, 1998
5. Bhagavan Das, Massage Therapy in Ayurveda, Concept publishing company, New Delhi, 1998
6. Bhavaprakash, Bhavaprakasha Samhita, Sanskrit –Marathi only, Raghuvanshi Publications, Pune, 1929
7. Charaka, Charaka Samhita, Varanasi, India, Chaukhamba Sanskrit Series, 1976
8. Dwight Byers, Better Health with Foot Reflexology, Ingham Publishing Inc.,U.S.; Rev Ed edition (Jun 2001)
9. Encyclopedia of Aromatherapy Massage and Yoga- Carole Mcgilvery, Jim Reed, Mira Mehta. Smith Mark Publishers, New York, USA, 1998
10. Frawley, David; Ranade, Subhash, Ayurveda Natures Medicine, Lotus Press, Twin Lakes, WI, 2001
11. Frawley, David, From the River of Heaven, Lotus Press, USA, Twin Lakes, WI, 1990
12. Harish, Johari, Ancient Indian Massage: Traditional Massage Techniques Based on the Ayurveda, Munshiram Manoharlal, India, January 2003
13. Nanal, M.P. and Garde, Mardanashastra, MP Nanal foundation, India, 1990
14. Pub Thornsons, Massage at your fingertips, Thorsons Publishers, Melbourne, Australia, 1984
15. Ranade, Subhash; Lele, Avinash, Panchakarma and Ayurvedic Massage, Published by International Academy of Ayurveda, Pune, India, 1997
16. Sushruta, Sushruta Samhita, Chaukhamba Sanskrit Series, Varanasi, India, 1981
17. Vatsyayana, The Kama Sutra of Vatsyayana: The Classic Burton Translation, Dover Publications, UK, July 21, 2006

RESOURCES

International Academy of Ayurveda

The International Academy of Ayurveda in Pune, India, whose chairman is Dr. Subhash Ranade and director is Dr. Avinash Lele, is one of the foremost institutions for training foreign students in India. It has complete facilities and programs for all levels of training from beginner to advanced, including special clinical instruction. It features a renowned faculty of Ayurvedic experts from throughout the world including Dr. Subhash Ranade, Dr. Avinash Lele, Dr. Abbas Qutab, Dr. Hans Rhyner, Dr. David Frawley and Mukunda Stiles. Pune itself is one of the most modern cities in India with a pleasant year round climate and easy airport access from Bombay (Mumbai), making it an ideal place in India to study.

The institute offers practical courses in Ayurveda, both basic and advanced. Special programs are available on the Fundamentals of Ayurveda, Pancha Karma, Ayurvedic Massage, Marma Therapy, Herbology and Clinical Studies. Programs are given July-August and November-January every year in classes of about ten students. Please register at least two months ahead of time to reserve your place.

The institute has its own line of books on Ayurveda in English by Dr. Ranade, Dr Lele, Dr. Frawley, and others, as well as other educational materials, (Ayurvedic CD-ROM) and herbal products, making it an important Ayurvedic resource center as well.

http://www.ayurveda-int.com
Dr. Subhash Ranade, Chairman
Email: sbranade@rediffmail.com

The Center for Vedic Medicine

The Center for Vedic Medicine is directed by David Freedman, Certified Ayurvedic Practitioner, and is involved in Vedic Medicine education, research and treatment. The Center for Vedic Medicine works with local, national and international medical professionals and educators involved in Vedic and other Oriental medicines. Education courses include Ayurvedic Medicine, Ayurvedic Massage, Yoga, Vastu (the effect of building and site design) and Jyotish (Indian Astrology). Courses are offered both online and in a live class format. Certification is granted upon course completion.

Future courses to include Tibetan medicine, Traditional Chinese Medicine and acupuncture.

Introductory courses and information are offered online free of charge. Electronic books are also available.

Center for Vedic Medicine
David Freedman, Director
www.vedicmd.com
1301-234th ST SW
Bothell, WA. 98021
425-485-0401
USA

Ayurveda Centers and Products

Aloha Ayurveda Academy
4504 Kukui Street
Suite 13
Kapaa HI, 96746
808-823-0994
www.hawaiiholisticmedicinecom

Dr. Suhas Kshirsagar, MD(Ayurveda),
Director
E-mail: drsuhashi@yahoocom
(808) 823-0994
Mobile: (808) 634-0050
Fax: (808) 823-0995

American Institute of Vedic Studies
PO Box 8357, Santa Fe NM 87504-8357
Dr. David Frawley (Pandit Vamadeva
Shastri), Director
Ph: 505-983-9385, Fax: 505-982-5807
Email: vedicinst@aol.com
www.vedanet.com

Aryavaidya Shala (Coimbatore)
136-137 Trichy Road
Coimbatore 641 045, T.N., India
ayurveda@vsnl.com
www.avpayurveda.com

Ateneo Veda Vyasa
Yoga Sadhana Ashram, 17041, Altare,
Savona, Italy
Tel/Fax - 0039-19-584838
E mail: ashram@tnt.it
Offers one year Ayurveda course.

Atreya Ayurved
Vd. M.Y. Lele Chowk,
Near Kamala Nehru Park
Erandawana, Pune. India 411004
Email: avilele@rediffmail.com

Australian College of Ayurvedic
Medicine
Dr. Frank Ros, Director
PO Box 322
Ingle Farm SA 5098
Australia
www.picknowl.com.au/homepages/
suchi-karma

Australian School of Ayurveda
Dr. Krishna Kumar, MD, FIIM
27 Blight Street
Ridleyton, South Australia 5008
Ph. 08-346-0631
Ayur-Veda AB
Box 78, 285 22 Markaryd
Esplanaden 2, Sweden
0433-104 90 (Phone)
0433-104 92 (Fax)
Email: info@ayur-veda.se

Ayurveda Academy
Dr. P.H. Kulkarni, President
36 Kothrud, Opp. Mhatoba Temple,
Pune 411 029, INDIA
Ph: 91-212-332130, Fax 91-212-363132
343933.
Email: ayurveda.academy@jwbbs.com

Ayurveda Clinic
Rajbharati, 367 Sahakar Nagar1,Pune
411 009,
Director- Dr. Sunanda Ranade
Tel/Fax 0091-20-4224427
E mail: snranade@hotmail.com
Offers Ayurvedic Counseling

Ayurveda for Radiant Health & Beauty
Ivy Amar
16 Espira Court
Santa Fe, NM 87505
Ph: 505-466-7662

Ayurvedic Academy & Wellness Center
819 NE 65th Street
Seattle, Washington USA 98115
Phone: (206) 729-9999
FAX: (206) 729-0164
www.ayurvedaonline.com

Ayurvedic Acupuncture Board of Ac-
creditation
19, Bowy Avenue, Enfield, SA, 5085,
Australia.
Director - Dr. Frank Ros
Tel./Fax 0061-08-83497303
E mail: suchi-Karma@picknow.com.au

Ayurvedic Institute of America.
561 Pilgrim Drive
Suite B
Foster City, California 94404
1-800-313-4372
650-341-8400
www.ayurvedainstitute.com

Ayurvedic Holistic Center
82A Bayville Ave.
Bayville, NY 11709
Swami Sadashiva Tirtha, Director
www.ayurvedahc.com

Ayurvedic Institute and Wellness Center
Dr. Vasant Lad, Director
11311 Menaul, NE
Albuquerque, NM 87112
Ph: 505-291-9698
www.ayurveda.com

California Association of Ayurvedic Medicine
www.ayurveda-caam.org

California College of Ayurveda
1117A East Main Street
Grass Valley, CA 95945
Ph: 530-274-9100
Two year state approved program in Ayurveda
www.ayurvedacollege.com
Email: info@ayurvedacollege.com

The Chopra Center
At La Costa Resort and Spa
Deepak Chopra and David Simon
7321 Estrella de Mar Road
Carlsbad CA 93009
Ph: 888-424-6772
www.chopra.com

John Douillard
Life Spa, Rejuvenation through Ayurveda
3065 Center Green Dr.
Boulder, CO 80301
Ph: 303-442-1164
www.LifeSpa.com

East West College of Herbalism
Hartswood, Marshgreen, Hartsfoeld,
Sussex TN7 4ET,U.K.
Tel.0044-1342-822312
E mail - EWCOLHERB@aol.com
Director- David and Sarah Holland
Offers 3 years Diploma course of Ayurveda.

European Institute of Vedic Studies
Atreya Smith, Director
Ceven Point N° 230
4 bis rue Taisson
30100 Ales, France
Ph: 33 (0) 680 61 79 96
Fax: 33-466-60-53-72
Ayurvedic training in Europe
Email: atreya@wanadoo.fr
www.atreya.com

Foundation for Health Promotion -
Fundacja Pomocy Zdrowiu
Ul.Belletiego 1, 01-022 Warsaw, Poland
Tel. 0048-22-6363401
Director-Zanna Kiesner
E mail - hacenter@kki.net.pl
Ganesha Institute
Pratichi Mathur, President
4898 El Camino Real, Suite 203
Los Altos CA 94022
Ph: 615-961-8316
www.healingmission.com

Himalayan Institute
RR1, Box 400
Honesdale, PA 18431
www.himalayaninstitute.org

Institute for Wholistic Education
3425 Patzke Lane
Racine, WI 53405 USA
(262) 619-1798
www.wholisticinstitute.org
Email: institute@infobuddhism.com

International Academy of Ayurveda
Chairman-Prof. Dr. Subhash Ranade
Director - Dr. Sunanda Ranade
www.ayurveda-int.com
Ph/Fax: 0091-20-24224427

International Ayurvedic Institute
11 Elm Street, Suite 103-105, Worcester,
MA,01609, U.S.A.
Tel. 001-508-775-3744
E mail: ayurveda@hotmail.com
Director - Dr. Abbas Qutab
Offers one year Ayurveda course

International Yoga Studies
Sandra Kozak, Director
692 Andrew Court, Benicia, CA 94510.
Ph: 707-745-5224
Email: IYSUSA@aol.com

Janaki Clinic and Panchakarma
Health Spa
Karve Nagar
S. No.72,

Near Spencers Daily
Pune - 411052, India.
Tel - +91-20-2-544-0386
Director - Dr. Bharati Lele.
E mail avilele@rediffmail.com
Offers basic and advance Ayurveda
Training, Panchakarma and counselling

Kaya Kalpa International
Dr. Raam Panday
111 Woodster Rd.
Satto, NY 10012

Kayakalpa
Sri Tatwamasi Dixit
22/2 Judge Jumbulingam Road
Off Radhakrishnan Salai, Mylapore
Chennai 600 004 India
www.mypandit.com

Life Impressions Institute
Attn: Donald Van Howten, Director
613 Kathryn Street
Santa Fe, NM 87501
Ph: 505-988-2627

Life in Balance Ayurvedic Rejuvenation
Center
418 N. 35th. St.
Seattle, WA. 98103
(206) 547-1330
www.ayurvedaseattle.com

Light on Ayurveda: Journal of Health
Genevieve Ryder, Editor/Publisher
418-77 Quinaquisset Avenue
Mashpee MA 02649
Ph: 508-477-4783
www.loaj.com

Light Institute of Ayurveda
Dr.'s Bryan & Light Miller
PO Box 35284
Sarasota, FL 34242
E-mail: earthess@aol.com
www.ayurvedichealings.com

Lotus Ayurvedic Center
4145 Clares St. Suite D
Capitola, CA 95010
Ph: 408-479-1667
www.lotusayurveda.com

Lotus Press
Dept. AMT, P. O. Box 325
Twin Lakes, WI 53181 USA
Ph: 262-889-8561
Fax: 262-889-8591
Email: lotuspress@lotuspress.com
Website: www.lotuspress.com
Publisher of books on Ayurveda,
Reiki, aromatherapy, energetic heal-
ing,
herbalism, alternative health and
U.S. editions of Sri Aurobindo's writ-
ings

National Association of Ayurvedic
Medicine
www.ayurvedic-association.org

National Institute of Ayurvedic
Medicine
584 Milltown Road
Brewster, NY 10509
Ph: 845-278-8700
www.niam.com
Email: niam@niam.com

Dr. Subhash Ranade
Rajbharati, 367 Sahakar Nagar 1
Pune 411 009, India
Email: sbranade@hotmail.com

Rocky Mountain Institute of Yoga
and Ayurveda
PO Box 1091
Boulder CO 80306
Ph: 303-499-2910
Email: rmiya@earthnet.net
www.rmiya.org

Salt Springs Spa
1460 North Beach Road
Salt Spring Island, B.C.
Canada V8K 1J4
1-800-665-0039
T (250) 537- 4111
F (250) 537-2939
www.saltspringspa.com

Sanskrit Sounds - Nicolai Bachman
PO Box 4352
Santa Fe, NM 87502
Email: shabda@earthlink.net
www.SanskritSounds.com

Sewa Akademie
Leutstettner Strasse 67/a,D-81477 Munich, Germany
Tel. 0049-89-7809777
E mail: ayurvedaseva@vsnl.com
Director-Dr. Hans Rhyner.

SKA Ayurveda
Via Aldo Moro 11, Pozzuolo, Martesana, Milano, 20060, Italy
Tel/Fax 0039-02-95358736
Director-Basilixa Querimint

Texas Yoga & Ayurveda Institute
Dr. Rob Francis, director
4008 Vista Rd. Bldg. B, Suite 201
Pasadena, Texas 77504
Ph: 713-941-9642
www.texasyoga.net

Vinayak Ayurveda Center
2509 Virginia NE, Suite D
Albuquerque, NM 87110
Ph: 505-296-6522
www.ayur.com

Vedic Cultural Fellowship
Howard Beckman, Director
HC 70 Box 620
Pecos NM 87552
Ph: 505-757-6194
www.vedicworld.org
Wise Earth School of Ayurveda
Maya Tiwari
(Sri Swamini Mayatitananda)
70 Canter Field Lane
Candler, NC 28715
www.wisearth.org

Ayurvedic Herbal Suppliers
Auroma International
Dept. AMT
PO Box 1008
Silver Lake, WI 53170
Ph: 262-889-8569
Fax: 262-889 8591
Email: auroma@lotuspress.com
Website: www.auroma.net
Importer and master distributor of Auroshikha Incense, Chandrika Ayurvedic Soap and Herbal Vedic Ayurvedic products.

AyurHerbal Corporation
PO Box 6390
Santa Fe, NM 87502
Ph: 262-889-8569
Manufacturer of Herbal Vedic Ayurvedic products.
Website: www.herbalvedic.com

Ayush Herbs, Inc.
10025 N.E. 4th Street
Bellevue, WA 98004
Ph: 800-925-1371

Banyan Botanicals
Traditional Ayurvedic Herbs
6705 Eagle Rock Ave N.E.
Albuquerque, NM 87113
Ph: 541-488-9525
1-800-953-6424
www.banyanbotanicals.com

Bazaar of India Imports
1810 University Avenue
Berkeley, CA 94703
Ph: 800-261-7662; 510-548-4110
www.bazaarofindia.com
Bio Veda
215 North Route 303
Congers, NY 10920-1726
Ph: 800-292-6002

Dr's Bryan and Light Miller
2017 Fiesta Drive
Sarasota, FL 34231
Ph: 941-929-0999
www.ayurvedichealers.com

Frontier Herbs
PO Box 229
Norway, IA 52318
Ph: 800-669-3275

HerbalVedic Products
PO Box 6390
Santa Fe, NM 87502
www.herbalvedic.com

Internatural
Dept. AMT
PO Box 489
Twin Lakes, WI 53181 USA
800-643-4221 (toll free order line)
262-889-8581 (office phone)
262-889-8591 (fax)
Email: internatural@lotuspress.com
www.internatural.com
Retail mail order and Internet re-seller of Ayurvedic products, essential oils, herbs, spices, supplements, herbal remedies, incense, books, yoga mats, supplies and videos.

Fern Life Center
710 Fifth Ave NW
Issaquah, WA 98027
Director- Keesha Ewers
425-391-3376
www.fernlifecenter.com

Lotus Brands, Inc.
Dept. AMT
PO Box 325
Twin Lakes, WI 53181
Ph: 262-889-8561
Fax: 262-889-8591
Email: lotusbrands@lotuspress.com
www.lotuspress.com

Lotus Herbs
1505 42nd Ave., Suite 19
Capitola, CA 95010
Ph: 408-479-1667
www.lotusayurveda.com

Kerala Ayurveda
Aptos, CA
Director- Dr. Suhas Kshirsagar
888-275-9103
www.ayurvedaonline.com

Lotus Light Enterprises
Dept. AMT
PO Box 1008
Silver Lake, WI 53170 USA
800-548-3824 (toll free order line)
262-889-8501 (office phone)
262-889-8591 (fax)
Email: lotuslight@lotuspress.com
www.lotuslight.com
Wholesale distributor of Ayurvedic
products, essential oils, herbs, spices,
supplements, herbal remedies, incense, books and other supplies. Must
supply
resale certificate number or practitioner license to obtain catalog of more
than 10,000 items.

Maharishi Ayurveda Products Interna-
tional
417 Bolton Road
PO Box 541
Lancaster, MA 01523
Info: 800-843-8332 Ext. 903
Order: 800-255-8332 Ext. 903

Om Organics
3245 Prairie Avenue, Suite A
Boulder, CO 80301
Ph: 888-550-VEDA
www.omorganics.com

Organic India
Affiliate of Om Organics
Indira Nager, Lucknow,
Uttar Pradesh, India 226016
www.organicindia.com

Planetary Formulations
PO Box 533
Soquel, CA 95073
Formulas by Dr. Michael Tierra
www.planetherbs.com

Tattva's Herbs
902 NE 65th St.
Suite D
Seattle, WA. 98115
206-380-2633
877-828-8824
Fax: 206-729-0565
www.tattvasherbs.com

Tri Health
Ayurvedic herbs and formulas from the
Kerala Ayurvedic Pharmacy.
Jeff Lindner, director, Kauai, Hawaii
Ph: 800-455-0770
Email: oilbath@aloha.net
www.oilbath.com

ABOUT THE AUTHORS

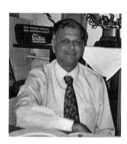

Dr. Subhash Ranade

Dr. Subhash Ranade is one of the foremost experts on Ayurveda. He is leading academician and physician in the field of Ayurveda. He is the author of 125 books on Ayurveda and Yoga. These books have been published in Marathi, Hindi, Malayalam, English, French, Czech, German, Greek, Italian, Japanese, Korean, Polish, Portuguese, Russian and Spanish languages.

He has worked as Prof. and Head, Dept. of Interdisciplinary School of Ayurveda and Prof. and Head, Dept. of Ayurveda Pune University and Principal of Ashtang Ayurveda College, Pune, India.

At present he is Chairman, International Academy of Ayurveda, Pune, (www.ayurved-int.com) and Honorary Dean, Kerala Ayurveda Academy, USA, (www.ayurvedaacademy.com). IAA imparts Ayurveda training and conducts basic courses, Advance courses, Ayurvedic Massage, Marma Therapy and Panchakarma for foreigners and Indians in Pune. Since 1996 IAA has trained more than 300 students from all over the world.

Professor Subhash Ranade has given many television interviews on Ayurveda, not only in India but also in USA, Poland, Italy, Germany, Brazil and Chili as well. He has also attended many International and National seminars on Ayurveda and Yoga. He has written hundreds of articles on Ayurveda and Yoga in various magazines and newspapers.

He has the honor of being visiting Professor to many Institutes in the United States like Kerala Ayurveda Academy Seattle, American Institute of Ayurveda, San Francisco, Los Angeles, Houston; Wellness center in Baltimore, USA; SEVA academy Munich and Veda Clinic, Charlottenhohe, Germany; SKA Ayurveda, Milan, Italy; School of Ayurvedic Culture, Barcelona, Spain; Body-Mind Health, Zurich, Swiss and Ultimate Health Center, Athens, Greece, Ayurvedic International Diffusing Association, Japan, Post Graduate Institute –Buenos Aires in Argentina, Yoga federation in Lisbon, Portugal and Israeli Center of Ayurveda, Broshim Campus, Tel Aviv.

His pioneering work in the field of CD ROM's like Dhanvantari and Marma and Massage have been whole-heartedly welcomed and highly appreciated by the Ayurvedic world. He has also helped to develop the first website on Ayurveda- www. saffronsoul.com

Since 1981, he has visited and conducted hundreds of Ayurveda courses for medical practitioners in Europe, Canada, USA, Brazil, Argentina, Chili and Japan.

Prof. Subhash Ranade, through his contacts world wide, was able to send more that 100 Ayurvedic Physician in various Countries like Poland, Spain, Italy, Israel, Swiss,

Germany, Philippines, Japan, USA and Singapore.

He was also appointed as Visitors Nominee at Banaras Hindu University by President of India for 3 years.

He has been chosen to be included in the website of Indian Autographs.

http://www.indianautographs.com/productdetail-209125.html

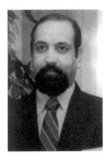

Dr. Rajan S. Rawat

Lecturer, Ashtanga Ayurveda College
2062, Sadashiv Peth, Pune 411,030
Member and Visiting Lecturer
International Academy of Ayurveda, Pune

Visits Abroad
Foundation for Health Promotion, Warszwa, Poland
Ateneo Veda Vyasa, Savona, Italy
SKA Ayurveda, Milano, Italy.

Courses Conducted
Have conducted many courses on Ayurveda and Yoga in India and Abroad
On Massage and Marma Therapy.

CD ROM
Contributed for the first CDROM on Ayurvedic massage and Marma Therapy.

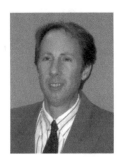

David Freedman
Editor

David Freedman is a Certified Ayurvedic Practitioner and is the director of the Center for Vedic Medicine, Bothell, Washington, USA. He is a graduate of the AYU Ayurvedic Academy where he studied under traditionally trained Ayurvedic doctors and surgeons including Dr. Subhash Ranade and Dr. Avinash Lele, both undergraduate and post graduate. He writes, teaches, practices and performs research in Oriental medicine including Ayurveda, Tibetan and Traditional Chinese Medicine.

Ayurveda
Nature's Medicine
by Dr. David Frawley & Dr. Subhash Ranade

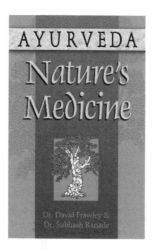

Ayurveda, Natures Medicine is an excellent introduction to the full field of Ayurvedic Medicine from diet and herbs to yoga and massage. It has a notable emphasis on practical self-care and daily life regimens that makes it helpful for everyone seeking health and wholeness. The book is an excellent primer for students beginning in the field and wanting to have a firm foundation to understand the entire system.

Trade Paper   ISBN 978-0-9149-5595-5   368 pp pb $19.95

Available at bookstores and natural food stores nationwide or order your copy directly by sending $19.95 plus $2.50 shipping/handling ($.75 s/h for each additional copy ordered at the same time) to:

Lotus Press, PO Box 325, Twin Lakes, WI 53181 USA
toll free order line: 800 824 6396 office phone: 262 889 8561
office fax: 262 889 2461 email: lotuspress@lotuspress.com
web site: www.lotuspress.com

Lotus Press is the publisher of a wide range of books and software in the field of alternative health, including Ayurveda, Chinese medicine, herbology, aromatherapy, Reiki and energetic healing modalities. Request our free book catalog.

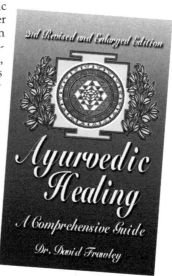

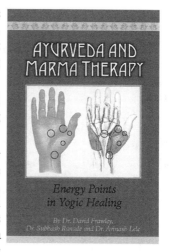

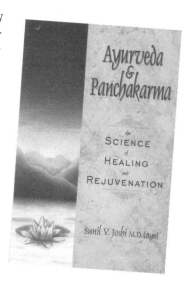